AF882222

The Glass Veil:
Seven Adventures in Wonderland

Art / Knowledge / Theory

Volume 2

Edited by
Suzanne Anker and Sabine Flach

PETER LANG
Bern · Berlin · Bruxelles · Frankfurt am Main · New York · Oxford · Wien

The Glass Veil: Seven Adventures in Wonderland

Suzanne Anker
Sabine Flach

PETER LANG
Bern · Berlin · Bruxelles · Frankfurt am Main · New York · Oxford · Wien

Bibliographic information published by die Deutsche Nationalbibliothek
Die Deutsche Nationalbibliothek lists this publication in the Deutsche Nationalbibliografie; detailed bibliographic data is available on the Internet at ‹http://dnb.d-nb.de›.

British Library Cataloguing-in-Publication Data: A catalogue record for this book is available from The British Library, Great Britain

Library of Congress Control Number: 2015930459

The editors and publishers gratefully acknowledge the permission granted to reproduce the copyright material in this book. Every effort has been made to trace copyright holders and to obtain their permission for the use of copyright material. The publisher apologizes for any errors or omissions in the above list and would be grateful if notified of any corrections that should be incorporated in future reprints or editions of this book.

Berliner Medizinhistorisches Museum der Charité

MEDICINSK MUSEION
Medicinens kultur - i går, i dag, i morgen

EMBL

ARTLABORATORYBERLIN

SVA NYC

艺术中心
V ART CENTER
复旦大学
上海视觉艺术学院

ISSN 2235-2759 pb.
ISBN 978-3-0343-1101-4 pb.

ISSN 2235-2767 eBook
ISBN 978-3-0351-0814-9 eBook

This publication has been peer reviewed.

© Peter Lang AG, International Academic Publishers, Bern 2015
Hochfeldstrasse 32, CH-3012 Bern, Switzerland
info@peterlang.com, www.peterlang.com

All rights reserved.
All parts of this publication are protected by copyright.
Any utilisation outside the strict limits of the copyright law, without the permission of the publisher, is forbidden and liable to prosecution.
This applies in particular to reproductions, translations, microfilming, and storage and processing in electronic retrieval systems.

Printed in Hungary

She generally gave herself very good advice
(though she very seldom followed it).

Lewis Carroll, *Alice's Adventures in Wonderland*

Table of Contents

Introduction 9

Acknowledgments 31

1. Essays

SUZANNE ANKER
Intimacy Unveiled 35

SABINE FLACH
Through the Looking Glass: Encounters with Suzanne Anker's Wonderlands 51

2. Dialogues

SUZANNE ANKER, SABINE FLACH

I The Glass Veil 71
II The Butterfly in the Brain / Rorschach 89
III Origins and Futures / Stem Cells 107
IV Laboratory Life / Genetic Seed Bank 121
V Biota / Carbon Collision of the Diamond Mind 137
VI Astroculture (Shelf Life) 153
VII Vanitas (in a Petri Dish) / Remote Sensing 167

Epilogue 187

3. Appendix

SUZANNE ANKER
Mendell's Meltdown 201
Errata/Erotica 205
Synthetic Abandon 211
Viruses and Pearls 215

Biographies 219

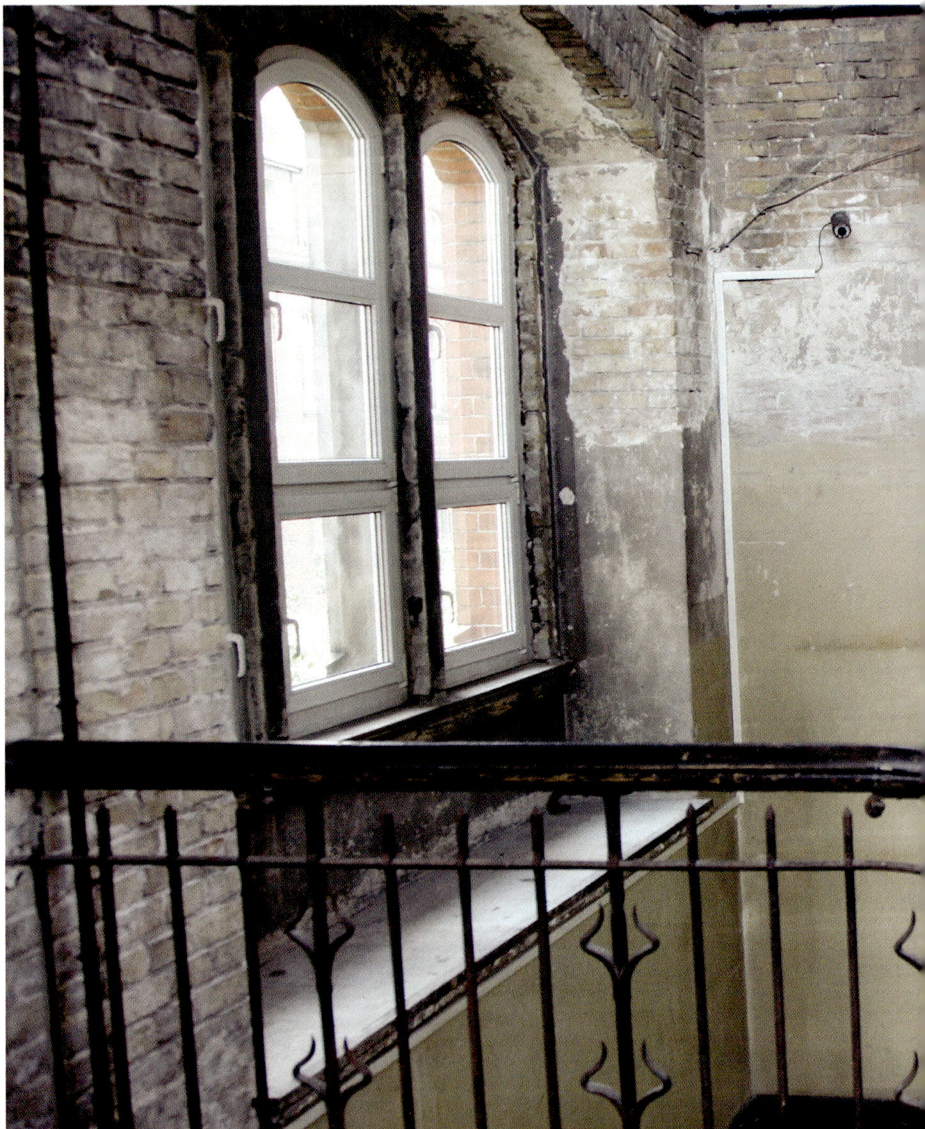

Figure 1. Suzanne Anker, *The Glass Veil (In and Out of Time)*, 2009.
Inkjet print on sintra, 76 x 96 in (193 x 243.84 cm). Installation view of *The Glass Veil* at Berliner Medizinhistorisches Museum der Charité, Berlin, Germany, 2009. Photograph by Suzanne Anker.

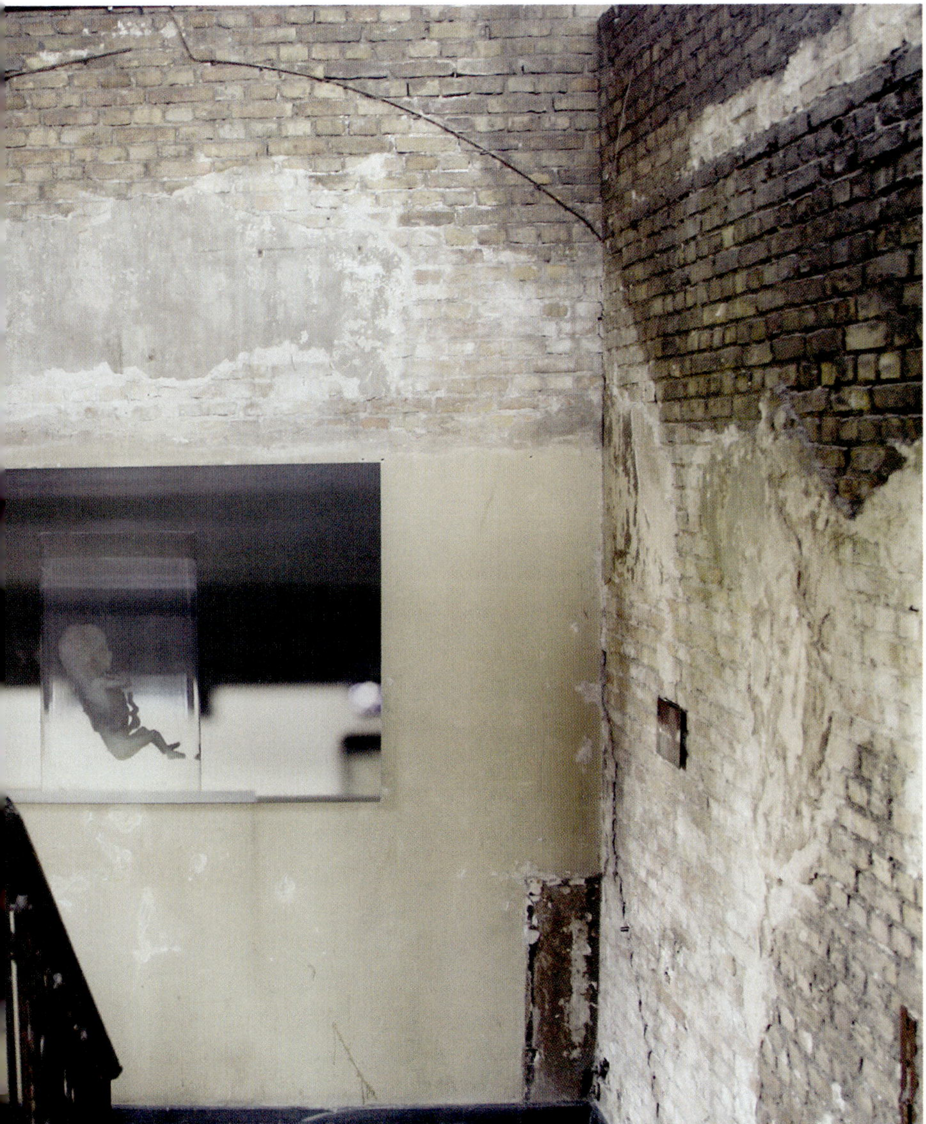

Figure 2. Suzanne Anker, *MRI Butterfly #4,* 2008.
Archival inkjet print on paper, 13 x 19 in (33 x 48 cm).

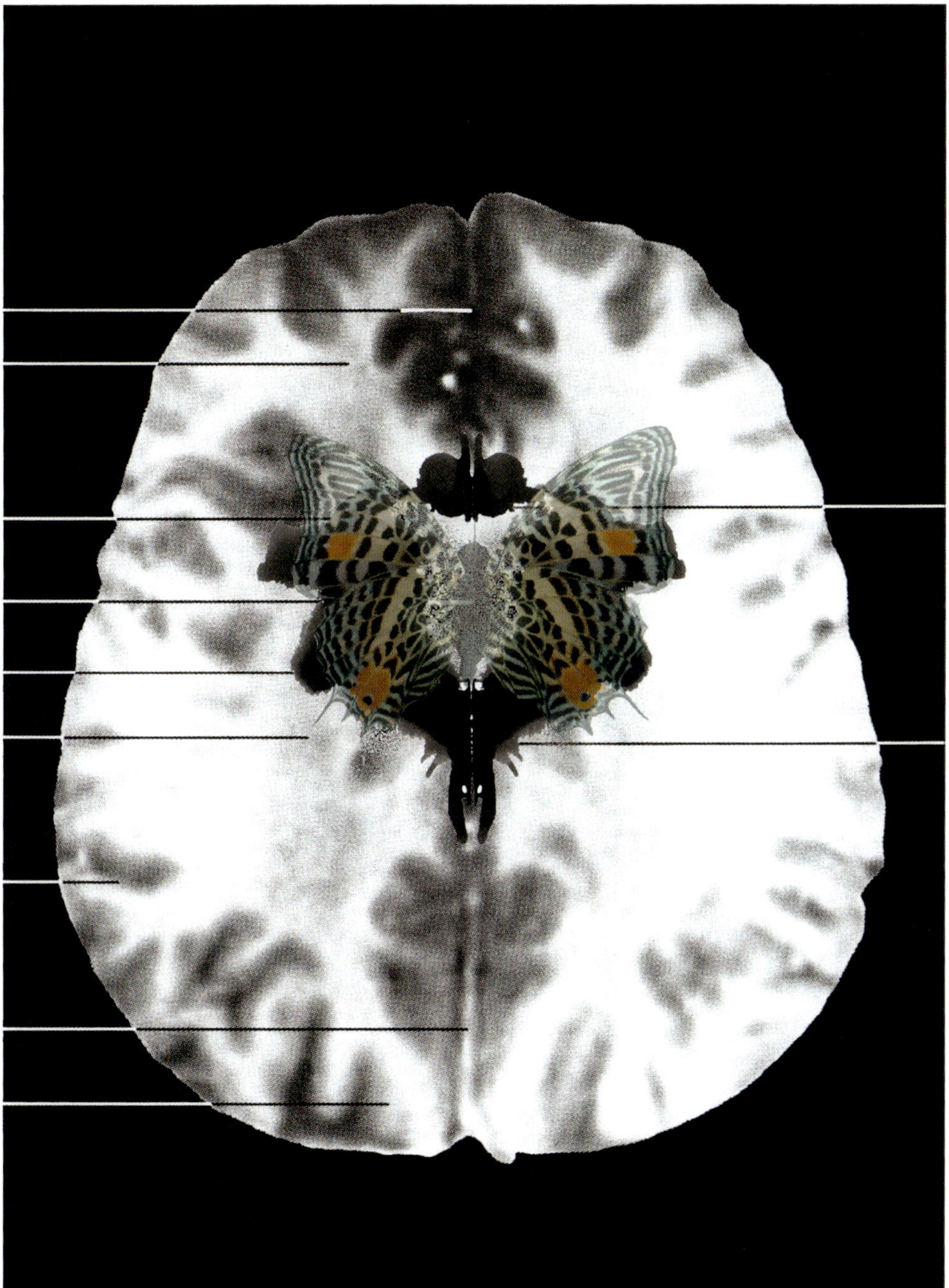

Figure 3. Suzanne Anker, *Origins and Futures*, 2004. Rapid prototype sculpture of plaster and resin, stainless steel, pyrite minerals, 96 x 96 in (243.84 x 243.84 cm). Installation view of *Golden Boy* at Universal Concepts Unlimited, New York City, 2004. Photograph by D. James Dee.

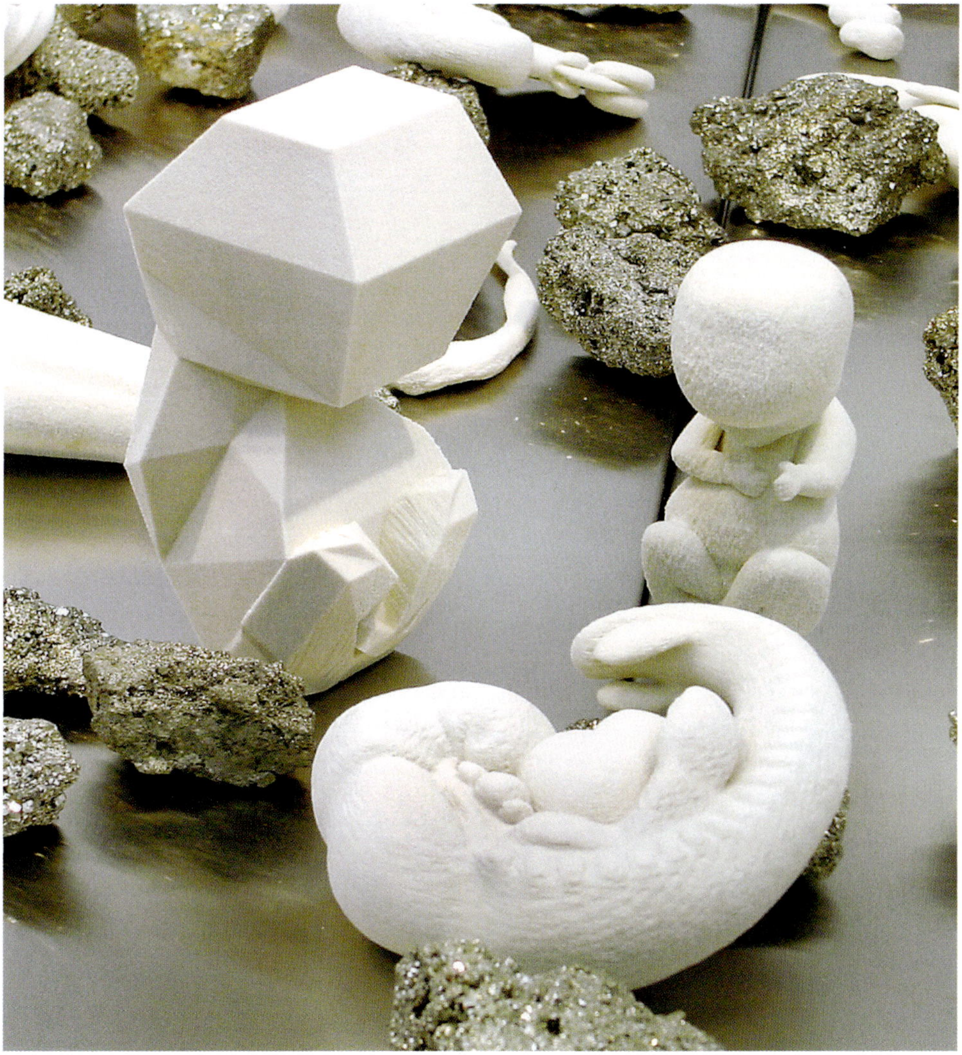

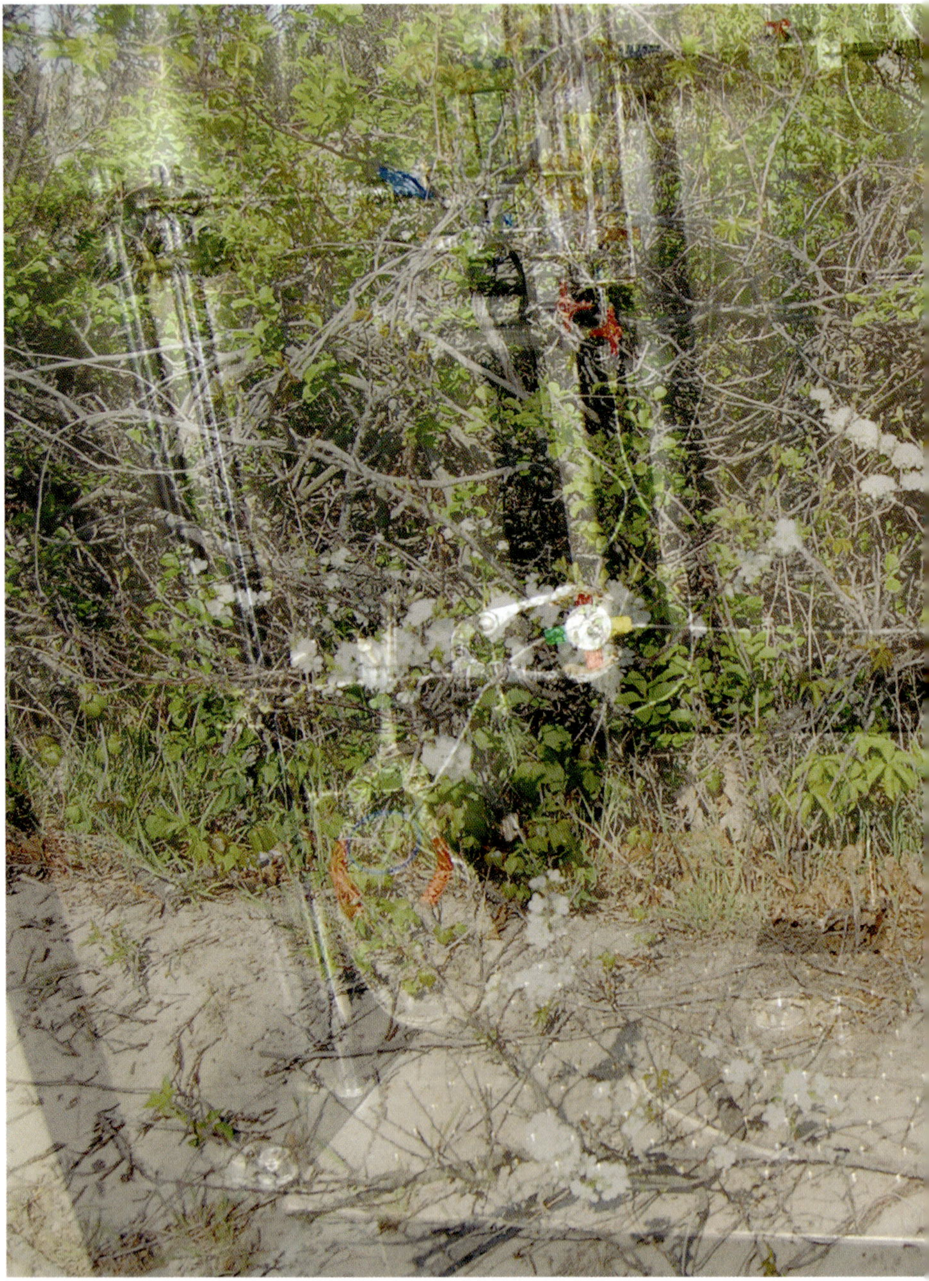

Figure 4. Suzanne Anker, *Laboratory Life (Bug Eye),* 2006.
Archival inkjet print on paper, 24 x 36 in (61 x 91.5 cm).

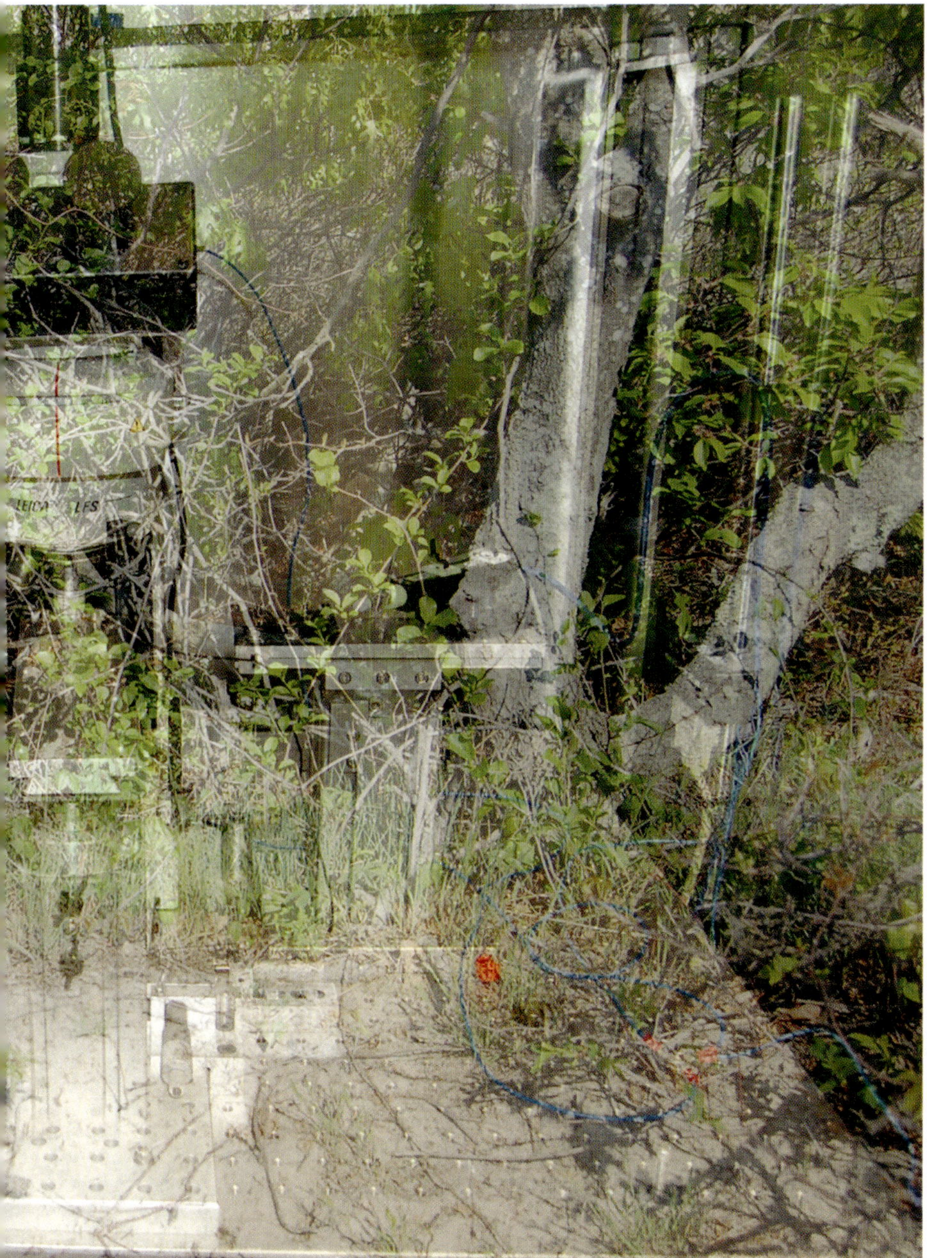

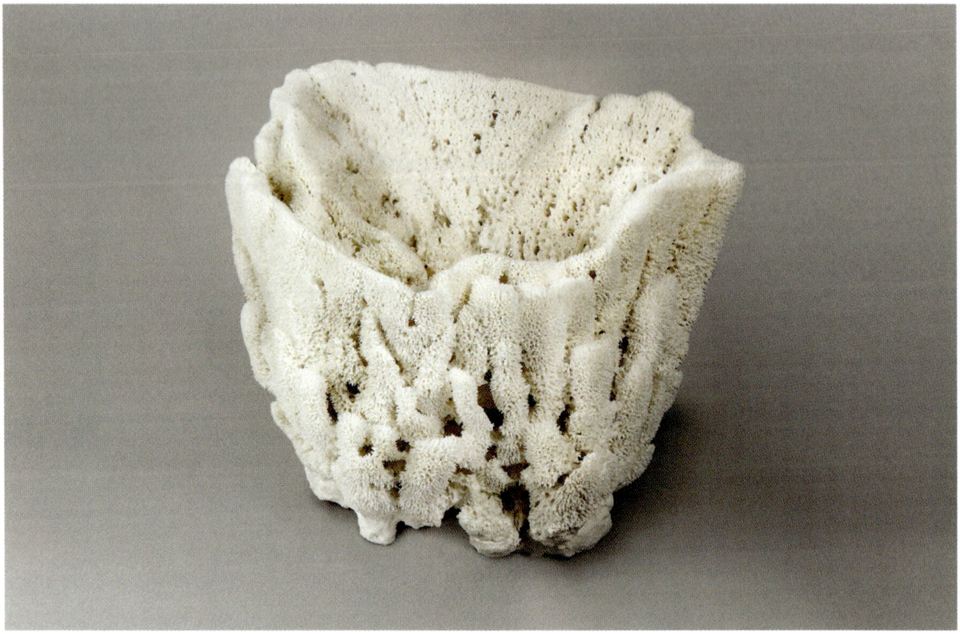

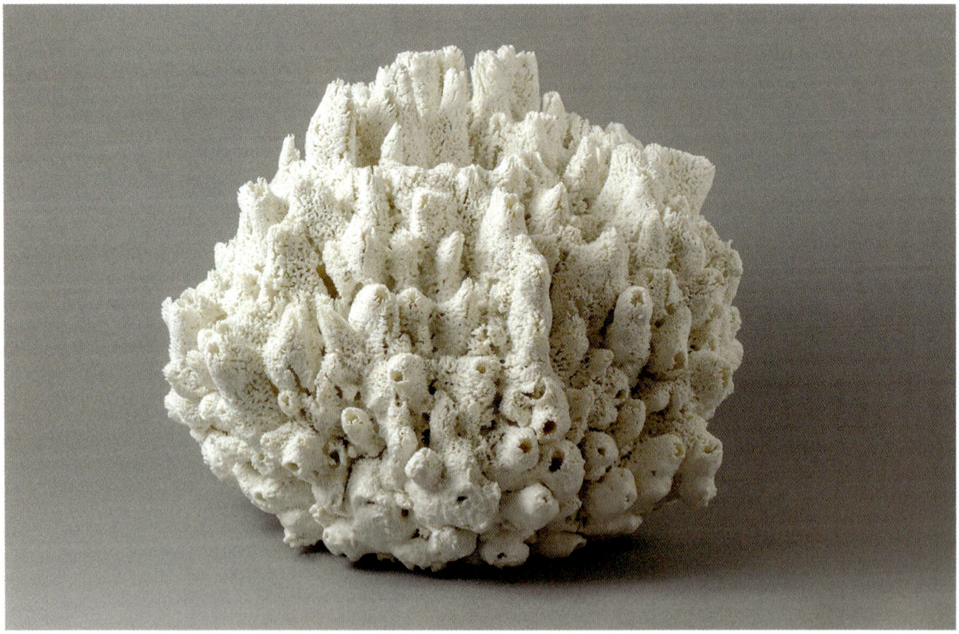

Figure 5. Top: Suzanne Anker, *Biota #3*, 2011. Porcelain, 5 x 8 x 7.5 in (12.7 x 20.3 x 19 cm). Bottom: Suzanne Anker, *Biota #108*, 2012. Porcelain, 12 x 11 x 8.5 in (30.5 x 28 x 21.6 cm). Photographs by Raul Valverde.

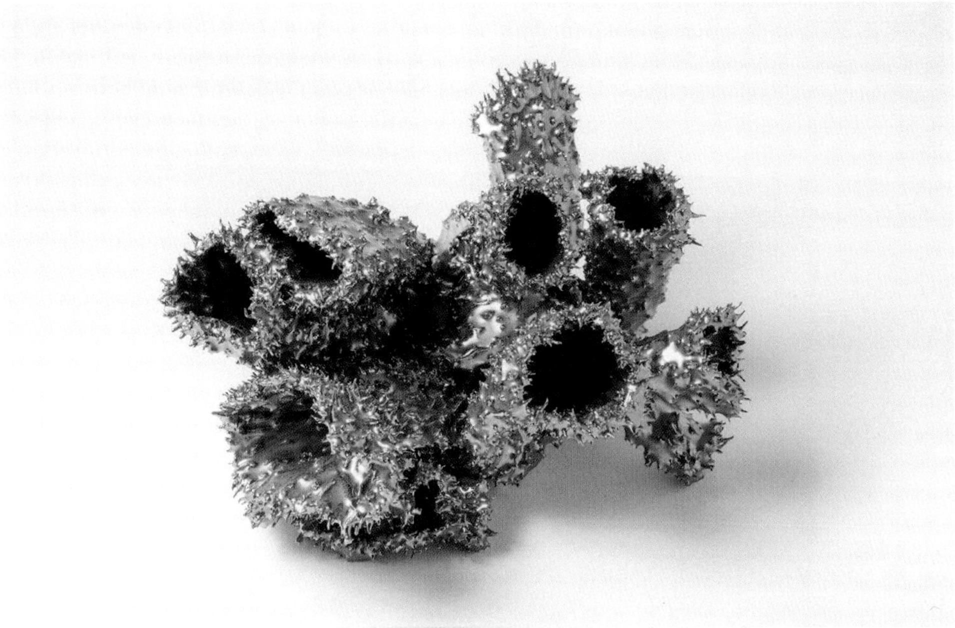

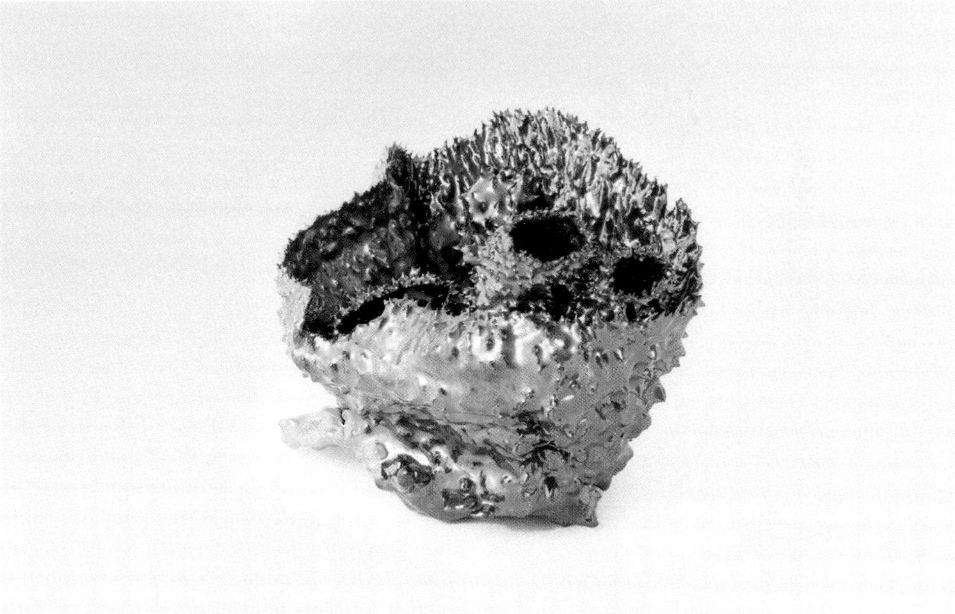

Figure 6. Top: Suzanne Anker, *Carbon Collision in the Diamond Mind #33,* 2014. Metallic-glazed porcelain sculpture, 6.5 x 5.5 x 4 in (16.5 x 14 x 10 cm). Bottom: Suzanne Anker, *Carbon Collision in the Diamond Mind #2,* 2014. Metallic-glazed porcelain scuplture, 8 x 5 x 5 in (20.3 x 12.7 x 12.7 cm). Photographs by Raul Valverde.

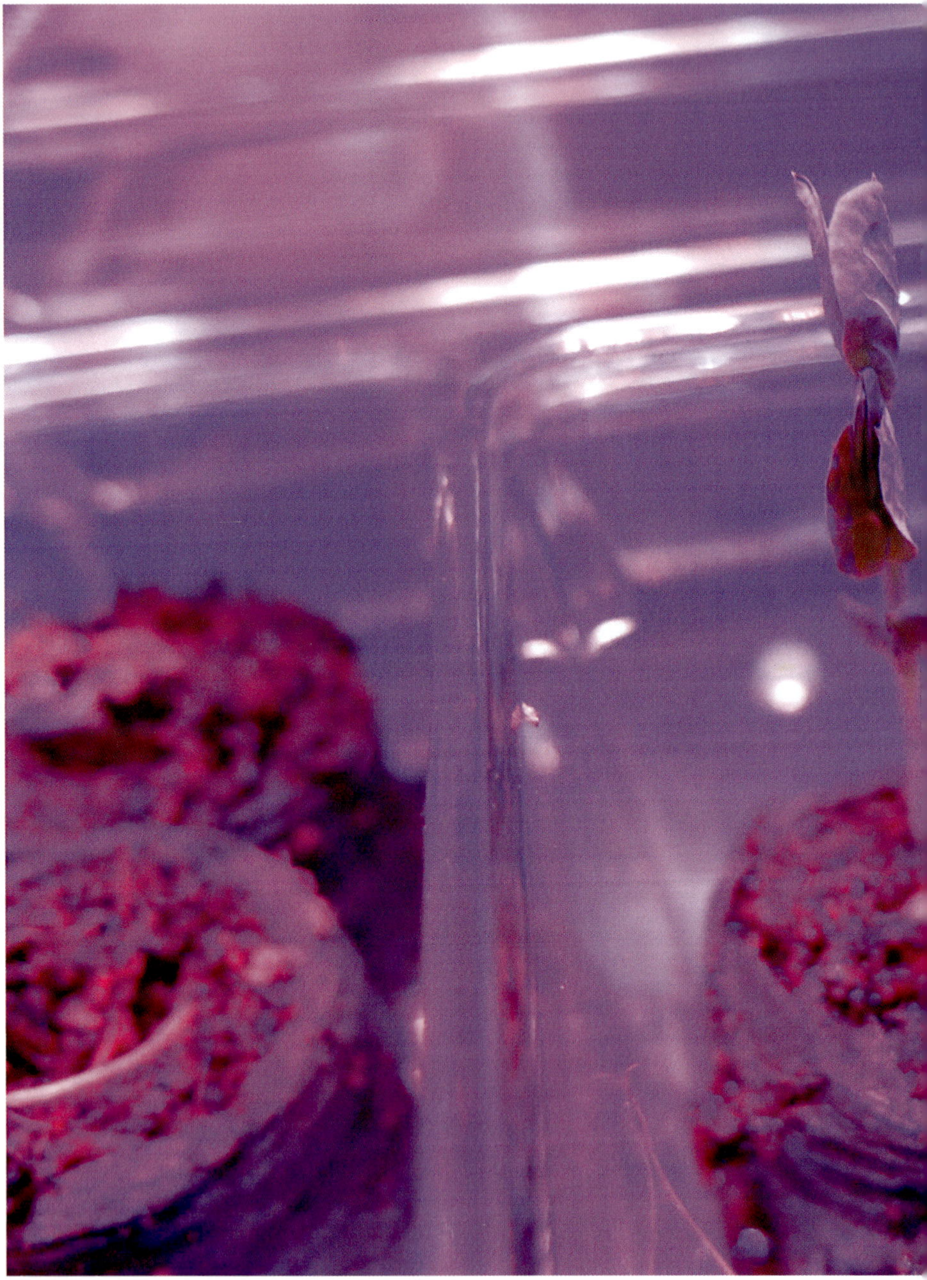

Figure 7. Suzanne Anker, *Astroculture (Shelf Life) II*, 2014. Installation view of *[macro]biologies II: organisms*, Art Laboratory, Berlin, 2014. Photograph by Suzanne Anker.

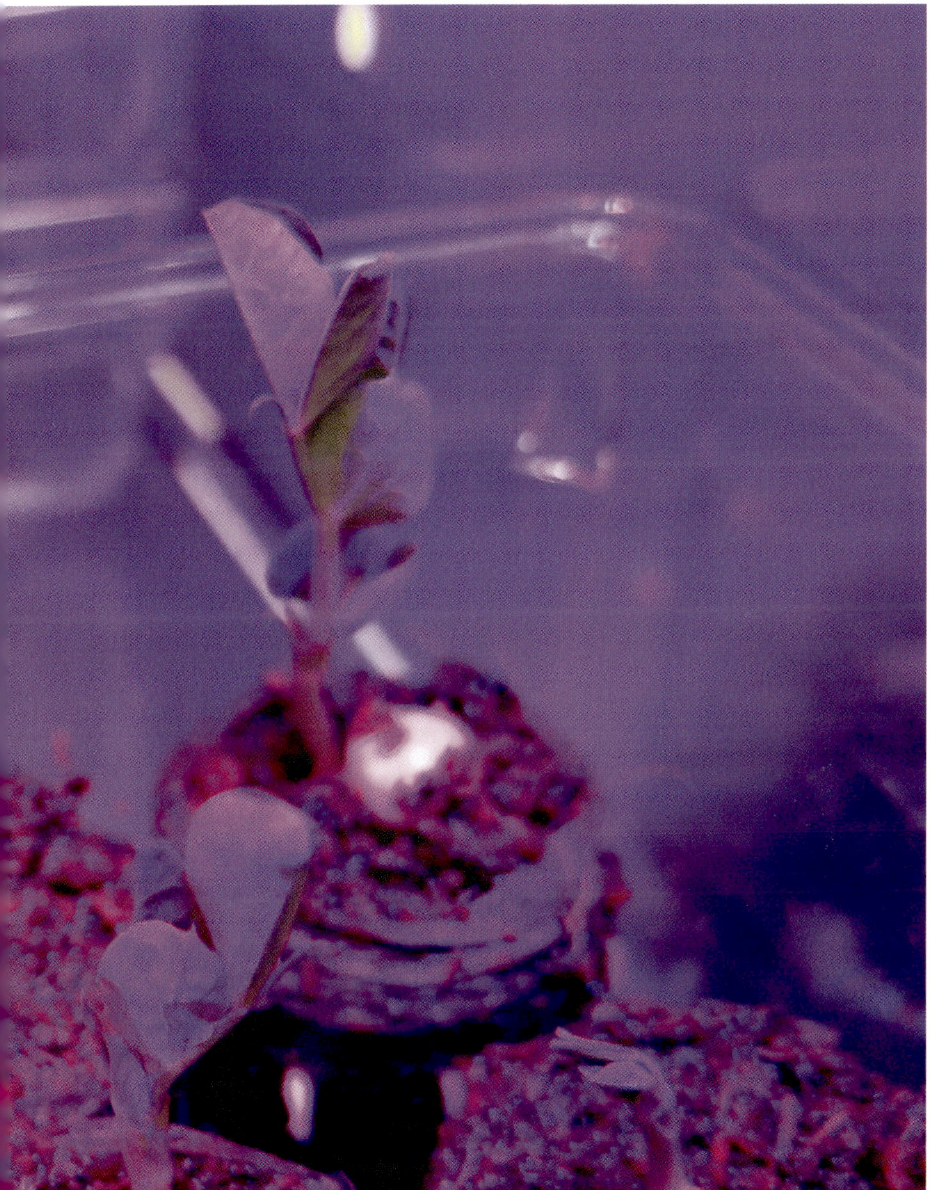

Figure 8. Suzanne Anker, *Vanitas (in a Petri Dish) #10*, 2013.
Archival inkjet print on paper, 44 x 44 in (111.7 x 111.7 cm).

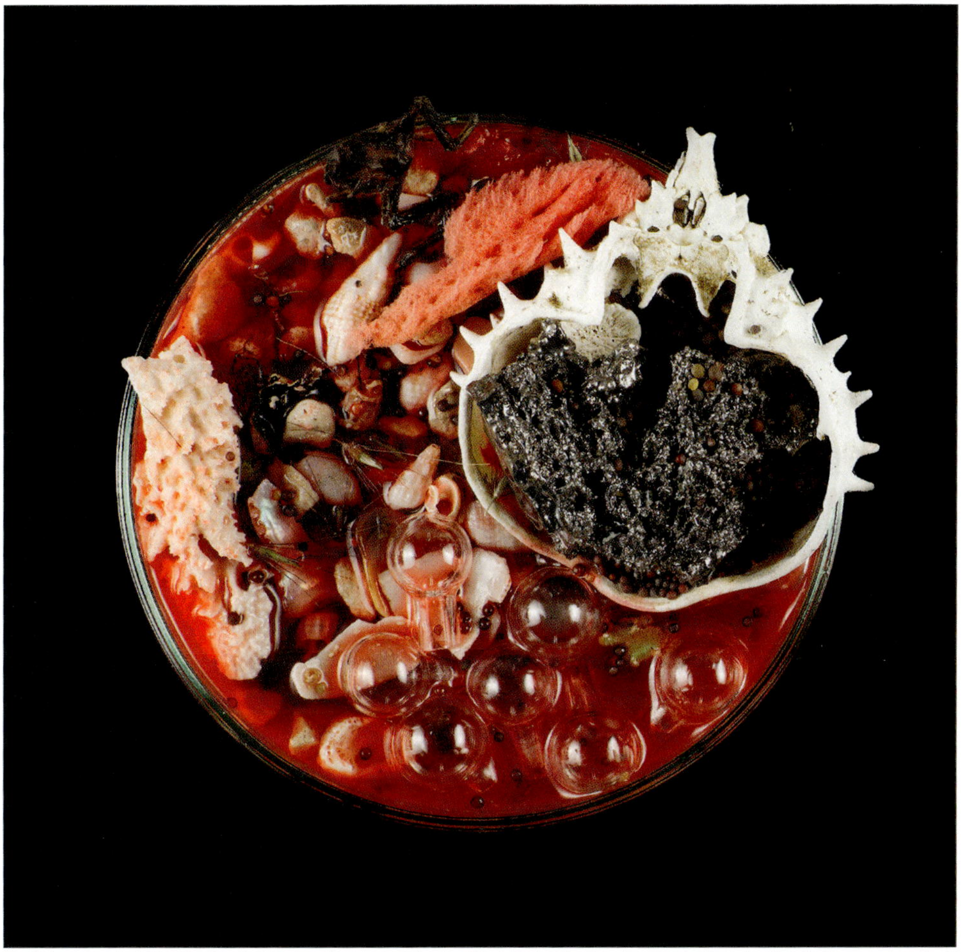

Introduction

The Glass Veil: Seven Adventures in Wonderland traces the coordinates, influences and investigations of Suzanne Anker's body of work from 2002 through 2014. The volume is not intended to be a comprehensive survey, but instead a dialogue between Suzanne Anker and Sabine Flach, an artist and art historian, respectively. Garnering a friendship that was sparked at an international conference of the Society for Literature, Science and the Arts (SLSA) in Amsterdam in 2006, we have continued to work together on various projects, of which this is one. Our evolving friendship has brought forth this book series *Art/Knowledge/Theory* that contains this volume. Other books in our series to date include *Embodied Fantasies: From Awe to Artifice* and Mika Elo and Miika Luoto's *Senses of Embodiment: Art, Technics, Media*. Future publications will include: *Frank Gillette: Axis of Observation.*

In this volume, we investigate the nature of perception and phenomenology as it applies to image-making processes inherent in the current intersections between the visual arts and biological sciences. As an interdisciplinary project, our own methodologies form a nexus underscored by those of art history, art theory, and philosophy. Connecting theory and practice, as we have learned from Gustave Flaubert's insightful short story *Bouvard et Pécuchet*, does not always line up congruently. In this fanciful story, the two protagonists retire from their positions as copy-clerks and move to the country to engage their passion – the pursuit of obtaining knowledge. No matter what they learn, theory's application to practice meets with failure, again creating a disparity between the two. However, it is this productive difference that is of significance to us. Like improvisational cooking or perceptual drawing or tableau photography, there are always variations and permutations involved in "making," even when the same set of materials or apparatuses are employed. Such subjective awareness and its intersubjective resonance is what guides our research.

An approach such as this one is central to what is comparable between thought and action. Does this dualistic model of the oft-cited "two cultures" remain a sustainable consideration or, alternately, has it become an historical myth? After all, the arts and the humanities have always worked empirically, just like the natural sciences. We can also clearly state that art can employ materials, media and techniques similar to those adapted for science and yet result in distinctly different outcomes. Works of art are not exhausted by the simple appropriation of "external" fields of knowledge such as biology and its allied technologies. In this regard they have capabilities that are not limited to mere critiques of ideology or subversive affirmations. These comparisons, or so we argue, presuppose a specific knowledge that is characteristically inherent in art, a knowledge that is irreducible. In other words, the genuine and productive accomplishments of art are the focus of this volume.

However, we also believe that affinities between these subjects are not the sole interest for these comparisons. By similarities we mean those trends in current debates revealing relationships between the arts, humanities and sciences. These considerations often rest on a problematic attempt to de-differentiate their distinct practices. Our methods and modes of inquiry do not seek to create a homogeneous space, but one of overlapping territories. Clichéd analogies comparing aesthetic elements such as beauty or creativity as aspects of each field have been overstated. As predominant as this comparison between art and science is, to attempt to link both fields in this manner is, in our view, extremely imprecise. Moreover, the practice of equating artistic products with scientific production renders the working methods in both fields strangely banal.

In the quest for pre-conceptual signs of creative activity, archetypes are formulated that predate the divided history of art and science and endeavor to reveal, in current discourses, the supposed unified aspirations of both. All too often art is ascribed as a humanistic activity that can make science more contemplative. In contrast to such problematic positions, we believe exchanges between the arts and sciences should initially focus on differences, not with the intention of drawing boundaries between the two fields, but with the goal of putting these distinctions to productive use. The objective is to formulate fundamental questions and marked solutions. After all, there is little sense in attempting to "define away" their methodological and epistemological disparities. Only then can we answer the question as to what epistemic status an artistic process is, in comparison to pure scientific research. What epistemic surplus might the arts presumedly have in correlation to scientific study? Our main goal is to specify the function of art asymmetrically, as art in relation to science, and to see art as something more than a mere medium of reflection.

As the title suggests, we have sought to invoke wonderland. In conceptual and imaginary terms, wonderland is a place where the extraordinary occurs. Far from utopian promises, wonderland is a morphing entity, sometimes even raucously out of control. From early investigations into the *Wunderkammer* to current discourses into speculative realism, wonder is an engine of fusion between lived experience and that which lies beyond. Conflating the ordinary with the supernatural has been evident in literature and film, especially since Mary Shelley's invocation of the classic *Frankenstein; or The Modern Prometheus* in 1818. Contemplating nature as a pantheistic form of godliness has engaged intellectuals from Spinoza to Emerson and Thoreau to name a few. Viewing nature as a data bank of resources yet to be untapped has, of course, met with repercussions that are severe and outlandishly frightening. From Chernobyl to global warming, we have witnessed the consequences of "unintended consequences." If wonderland is to be invoked, it is this time as a reclamation project, a reordering reverence for life's unbounded quarry, but not without stupendous awe for its Janus-faced darker side.

The influence of the biological sciences on contemporary art continues its journey from the Paleolithic eruption of human/animal hybrids through periods of the grotesque and Romanticism and beyond, where nature's *imprimatur* moves from representation to materiality to modernism and beyond. Such an overarching idiom is one that carries with it the enormity of discourses beginning, at least, with Aristotle. Present day contributors to these discussions are numerous and include Barbara Maria Stafford, Martin Kemp, Donna Haraway, Bruno Latour, Sarah Franklin, Vilém Flusser among others. It is within this vein of articulation that we direct our persuasions.

This ongoing dialogue also includes discourses in Bio Art, Bio Design and Bio Architecture. William Myers's recent text *BioDesign: Nature + Science + Creativity*, published by the Museum of Modern Art in New York City in 2012, broadens this concept. In addition, leading-edge advances in three-dimensional software programs contribute to visualization techniques fundamental to the output of novel materials and imaginary forms. A search in DIY Biology, a grassroots movement similar to computer hacking in the 1990s, is responsible for the start-ups of many community bio-labs internationally. Many of these projects and manifestations look towards the cell as the underlying ore where the potential for altering life is most pronounced. Current investigations into synthetic biology represent a significant change in how life itself can be conceptualized and even reconfigured.

Sabine Flach's essay, *Through the Looking Glass: Encounters with Suzanne Anker's Wonderlands* begins this volume. Flach analyzes the uniqueness of Anker's artistic productions by pointing, at once, to the dual nature of images, advanced technological tools, contemporary aesthetic strategies and cross-media explorations.[1] Her philosophical inquiry revisits, from a phenomenological perspective, the ideas of Maurice Merleau-Ponty and Edmund Husserl as well as

1 See also: *WissensKünste. Artistic knowledge and the art to know*, edited together with Sigrid Weigel, Weimar 2012 and *Sensing Senses. Die WissensKünste der Avantgarden. Künstlerische Theorie und Praxis zwischen Wahrnehmungswissenschaft, Kunst und Medien. 1915–1930* forthcoming 2015. Through these books and numerous articles and her first collaboration with a museum – Hamburger Bahnhof, Museum für Gegenwart, Berlin from 2000 to 2005 – Flach developed a methodological approach to encounter the specific knowledge of artistic production and to compare and analyze it.

more recent approaches to embodiment theories. Flach positions Anker's artwork as a site of practices and mental experiments, as an intermediary realm that interacts with elegance and ease *between* art and science *as* art. As a consequence, the paths, actions, methods and practices preceding the concrete results assume greater importance. The goal is to scrutinize the processes of production besides the actual results. Flach underlines that both process and product are embedded in the signification of traces left in images. Anker's images and sculptural objects are at the center of her attention which encapsulate these ideas in material forms. In her field of knowledge, it must be said that pictorial concepts do not reduce her art to a mere retinal representation, but perform a double function, namely, as a material substrate and a mental image.

In this sense, these images become figures of knowledge. They represent an historical index as a signature of visual thought. The image is always a process of compression in which past and present impressions combine. In other words, what is of consequence are the divergent ways of dealing with both images and the various types and media of pictorial representations.

The epistemological gain that results from studying the knowledge in the arts clearly lies in the experimental questioning of artistic as well as scientific concepts and procedures. This examination brings to light the not-yet-realized connections and hidden or invisible complexities, the zones of non-knowledge enclosed in knowledge as being a significant part of it. Her practice reveals them as blind spots and omissions, spaces of negation and the unconscious, which all form the counterpart to knowledge and give it its contours and depth. Flach's interest is to show that Anker's art is not concerned with becoming an ideologue or admonisher of ethical and practical questions, but rather with formulating appropriate queries to cope with the complexity of current aesthetic problematics and the way they filter out into the world.

In Anker's introductory text, *Intimacy Unveiled*, she briefly outlines both her artistic sources and her access to institutional archives, sites and objects. Her travels over the last ten years have opened up novel resources for her work. As an aspect of art's current globalized position, Anker's participation in exhibitions and symposiums in the Americas, Europe and Asia has made her a "frequent flyer." Unlike her other texts which range in tone and content from the staunchly analytic to the opinionated editorial, this text is more personal and diaristic. Citing visits to Auschwitz-Birkenau in Poland, the Marine Biological Laboratory in Woods Hole, Massachusetts, the D'Arcy Thompson Zoology Museum in Dundee, Scotland and an expert meeting pertaining to the subject of the fetus at Cambridge University in the United Kingdom, Anker sets up an ongoing travelogue of her experiences and layered thoughts.

This volume is divided into seven dialogues, recounting particular sets of Anker's work in the visual arts. In the first Dialogue, *The Glass Veil*, photographs created from the collections of the Museum Vrolik in Amsterdam, the Netherlands, the Medical Museion in Copenhagen, Denmark and the Medizinhistorisches Museum der Charité in Berlin, Germany are highlighted (fig. 1, pp. 8-9). All of these images bring forth somatic reactions in viewers as they are confronted in each case with human remains. These images point to myriad cultural questions concerning consent, disease, social mores, laboratory practices and, of course, mortality.

Dialogue II, *The Butterfly in the Brain*, moves on to engage art in relation to the neurosciences. Exploring the brain and its attendant metaphorical associations, this chapter illustrates some of the ways in which the brain and its nervous system can be visualized. Referring to MRI brain scans and Rorschach tests as devices explicating brain morphology and psychologically driven projective techniques, Anker's work, in a variety of mediums, cites the brain as an illusive force (fig. 2, p. 11).

Dialogue III, *Origins and Futures,* comments on theories related to the origin of life and its subsequent transformative status into a commodity. From cells to tissues to organs to whole bodies themselves – all have become fungible goods to be dissected, duplicated, marketed and patented. What bio-ethical issues emerge with regard to the manipulation and commercialization of living forms? Citing A.G. Cairns-Smith's theory on the origin of life, Anker reworks this hypothesis into a sculptural installation accompanied by digitally derived prints (fig. 3, p. 13).

In Dialogue IV, *Laboratory Life* and *Genetic Seed Bank* are onsite photographs of scientific laboratories: the Imperial Blast Biomechanical & Biophysics Laboratory at Imperial College in London, the European Molecular Biological Laboratory (EMBL) in Rome, and Mote Tropical Research Laboratory in the Florida Keys in the United States. In the former series, scientific apparatuses are overlaid with images of nature, man-made gardens, wild floral outcrops and their like (fig. 4, pp. 14-15). In the latter, laboratory photographs of coral in specially fabricated tanks occupy the field. This discussion looks at the ways in which nature has become a construction.

Dialogue V, *Biota* (fig. 5, p. 16) and *Carbon Collision of the Diamond Mind* (fig. 6, p. 17), moves biological metaphors into geological zones. While *Biota* is an ode to the sponge as the first multicellular organism on earth, *Carbon Collision of the Diamond Mind* invokes astrobiology and outer space as a trove of untapped resources.

Dialogue VI, *Astroculture (Shelf Life)*, a term employed by NASA apropos of their development of growing plants in space, is the impetus behind this series of work. Using live plants under controlled lighting sources, Anker's vegetables are grown in dark apartments or buildings without insecticides. Here nature is brought inside, protected in a sense by an artificial womb, a living *Wunderkammer* (fig. 7, pp. 18-19). Each seed is started in a small peat pod and sprouts within a few days. Such fascination is evident as the seeds grow towards maturity, first as a plant, then as a flower and finally as a fruit.

In Dialogue VII, *Vanitas (in a Petri Dish)* and *Remote Sensing* employ the Petri dish as a cultural icon. Relating current discourses into the manipulation of matter to concerns in 17th and 18th century Western paintings, *Vanitas (in a Petri Dish)* brings to the fore ethical arguments concerning biotech practices in the 21st century (fig. 8, p. 21). *Remote Sensing*, a series of rapid prototype sculptures appearing as micro landscapes, takes its cue from the disastrous impacts of toxicity and war. Remote sensing, a term derived from satellite technology, employs computer-generated data to assess geographical areas that are too problematic or dangerous for human intervention.

Finally, the Epilogue is a summation of thoughts and after-thoughts expressed in this volume. It concentrates on concepts inherent in defining what is being referred to as Bio Art, an international art movement involved with living matter and its advanced technological surround. In the Appendix are several early essays by Suzanne Anker written in conjunction with various art exhibitions in the United States and abroad: *Synthetic Abandon*, *Erratica/Erotica*, *Mendell's Meltdown* and *Viruses and Pearls,* authored between 1992 and 1993. They document Anker's initial interest in art and genetics. These brief essays are antecedent to the appearance of the first draft of the Human Genome in 2000, exemplifying her early forays into writing about these "life-altering" intersections.

References

Bernhard, Dotzler. "Explorationen. Literaturforschung und die Geschichte des Wissens und der Wissenschaften." In *Berichte und Abhandlungen. Volume 9*, 311-327. Berlin: Berlin-Brandenburgische Akademie der Wissenschaften, 2002.

Flach, Sabine and Sigrid Weigel. *Wissens Kuenste. Artistic knowledge and the art to know*, Weimar: VDG, 2012.

Flach, Sabine: *Sensing Senses. Die WissensKünste der Avantgarden. Künstlerische Theorie und Praxis zwischen Wahrnehmungswissenschaft, Kunst und Medien. 1915–1930*. In preparation, 2015.

Flaubert, Gustave, and Edouard Maynial. *Bouvard et Pécuchet: oeuvre posthume*. Paris: Garnier, 1965.

Myers, William. *Bio Design: Nature, Science, Creativity*. New York: Museum of Modern Art, 2012.

Shelley, Mary Wollstonecraft, Percy Bysshe Shelley, and Charles E. Robinson. *Frank-*

enstein, or, The Modern Prometheus: The Original Two-Volume Novel of 1816-1817 from the Bodleian Library Manuscripts. New York: Vintage Books, 2009.

List of Illustrations

Fig. 1: Suzanne Anker, *The Glass Veil (In and Out of Time)*, 2009. Inkjet print on sintra, 76 x 96 in (193 x 243.84 cm). Installation view of *The Glass Veil* at Berliner Medizinhistorisches Museum der Charité, Berlin, Germany, 2009. Photograph by Suzanne Anker.
Fig. 2: Suzanne Anker, *MRI Butterfly #4,* 2008. Archival inkjet print on paper, 13 x 19 in (33 x 48 cm).
Fig. 3: Suzanne Anker, *Origins and Futures*, 2004. Rapid prototype sculpture of plaster and resin, stainless steel, pyrite minerals. 96 x 96 in (243.84 x 243.84 cm). Installation view of *Golden Boy* at Universal Concepts Unlimited, New York City, 2004. Photograph by D. James Dee.
Fig. 4: Suzanne Anker, *Laboratory Life (Bug Eye),* 2006. Archival inkjet print on paper, 24 x 36 in (61 x 91.5 cm).
Fig. 5: Top: Suzanne Anker, *Biota #3*, 2011. Porcelain, 5 x 8 x 7.5 in (12.7 x 20.3 x 19 cm). Bottom: Suzanne Anker, *Biota #108*, 2012. Porcelain, 12 x 11 x 8.5 in (30.5 x 28 x 21.6 cm). Photographs by Raul Valverde.
Fig. 6: Top: Suzanne Anker, *Carbon Collision in the Diamond Mind #33,* 2014. Metallic-glazed porcelain sculpture, 6.5 x 5.5 x 4 in (16.5 x 14 x 10 cm). Bottom: Suzanne Anker, *Carbon Collision in the Diamond Mind #2,* 2014. Metallic-glazed porcelain sculpture, 8 x 5 x 5 in (20.3 x 12.7 x 12.7 cm). Photographs by Raul Valverde.
Fig. 7: Suzanne Anker, *Astroculture (Shelf Life) II*, 2014. Installation view of *[macro]biologies II: organisms*, Art Laboratory, Berlin, 2014. Photograph by Suzanne Anker.
Fig. 8: Suzanne Anker, *Vanitas (in a Petri Dish) #10*, 2013. Archival inkjet print on paper, 44 x 44 in (111.7 x 111.7 cm).

Acknowledgments

The Glass Veil: Seven Adventures in Wonderland required the expertise of many accomplished and gracious people, whom I wish to thank. Raul Valverde, Henry Sanchez and Tim Deussen for their photographic prowess and diligent work. To my dear friend and colleague, Giovanni Frazzetto, with whom I have shared many intriguing laboratory and writing experiences. To David Sarma for his skills in animation. To Tarah Rhoda, my assistant extraordinaire, whose dedication is unmatched. To Amy Stienbarger, for her help with my porcelain sculptures and Luis Navarro for his expertise in 3D printing. To Richard Dempsey for his attention to detail with regard to glazing and silver-leaf. To Frank Gillette for his succinct and elegant editing skills. To Gloria Houng for her superb technical editing. To Lisa Jeschke for her German/English translation. To Raul Valverde again, for his excellent design of this book and its associated graphic conceptions. To Dr. Kevan Main of the Mote Marine Laboratory for granting me access to the Tropical Research Center in the Florida Keys. To Thomas Söderqvist of the Medical Museion in Copenhagen, Thomas Schnalke of the Medizinhistorisches Museum der Charité in Berlin, and to Regine Rapp and Chris de Lutz from Art Laboratory Berlin for engaging with novel ideas and exhibiting art work that elucidates the relevant issues impacting the natural world. To Chiara Donelli for taking such good care of my sprouting seedlings in Berlin. To Sebastian Cocioba of New York Botanics for teaching me how to tissue culture African Violets. To Joseph DeGiorgis and the Marine Biological Laboratory at Woods Hole in Massachusetts for mentoring me on the principles of aquatic life forms. To Dan Fairbanks for organizing many of the images for this text as an aide-de-camp. To Sarah Franklin, for introducing me to her anthropological approach in researching blastocysts in Petri dishes and the inner workings of in vitro reproductive technologies. To Deborah and William Colton for their support and belief in my work. To Wolf-Dieter Stoeffelmeier and Marian Ziola, for their early support of my work at Universal Concepts Unlimited in NYC. To Papo Colo and the memory of Jeanette Ingberman for exhibiting my art and science related projects at their alternative gallery space in NYC, Exit Art. To art historian Sabine Flach for her engagement with my work and her philosophically stimulating inspiring thoughts. To my precious family – Frank Gillette my spouse equivalent, my daughter Jocelyn Anker and my amazing granddaughter Esme Anker Townsend for granting me time away from home to pursue my adventures. To President David Rhodes, Executive Vice President Anthony Rhodes and Provost Jeff Nesin for allowing me to develop my experimental pedagogical practices at the School of Visual Arts in New York City.

1. Essays

Intimacy Unveiled

SUZANNE ANKER

Works of art are fragile substances, sometimes materially incarnated and at other times mere actions, or even ephemeral thoughts. To think and more profoundly to embody this form of magical thinking is life's creative potential and nagging imposition. Obsessionally driven to engage in the process of what comes next, the artist, like the gymnast, summons his powers of concentration and moves center stage into the zone. Even in private, such obliqueness to life carries with it a special spatial coordinate in which failure is not an option. I am thinking about Käthe Kollwitz as she describes in her writings the loss of her son and the ways in which her art became a substitute for life. She speaks of her journey of driven desire, internally apprehended as a withdrawal from life itself. To embark upon a life filled with stops-and-starts, is not particular to artists of a certain sort. But some artists must account for time spent, removed from the practicalities of life, while others engage themselves in the high-stake returns of artist-as-entrepreneur. Like sumo wrestlers sitting in economy airplane seats, some artists have built-in mutability meters and can adjust as necessary in playing art world monopoly. Others are not well suited for such approaches. Ascetic, ravished, egomaniacal, insecure or eccentric are some of the words to describe an artist's states of being.

Over the past number of years I have pursued projects which have brought me closer to the idea that art is a form of social thought. Apportioned between philosophy, sociology and art historical rumination, these persuasions have entered territories ranging from taboo to beauty. In such adventures, and there have been many more that remain private, my work has consistently explored the boundaries between received ideas, experimental longings and the wonders of the natural order. That is not to say that nature rules without tacit malevolence, as one creature devours another in order to exist, nature's food chain is an inbred pattern of an extant code.[1] Notwithstanding that environmental factors can be ignored, certain hardwired traits have no redemption, even as part of nature's cycle.

The following chapters bring the reader closer to where I have been, my flights of fancy and my international wandering. Criss-crossing the Atlantic has

1 At the School of Visual Art's Bio Art Lab in New York City, several aquatic species, including the African clawed Xenopus frog are contained within aquariums. The Lab started out with many of these frogs but our numbers have decreased for a variety of reasons. The most shocking aspect of this reduction came about through their own cannibalistic acts, as one frog devoured another. See http://bioart.sva.edu for more information.

become commonplace, thus creating an expanded network of colleagues, institutions, and landscapes. In addition I have had extraordinary access to objects of various pedigree and dispensation, which have imprinted their canonical history and circumstance on my thoughts.

From medical museums to aquatic research centers, from neurological institutes to genetic laboratories, from botanical gardens to food markets, these sites have been incorporated into my data bank of research tools. Add to the mix access to new technologies and the construction of the School of Visual Art's Bio Art Laboratory[2] (figs. 9-11). I have within reach the raw materials for expanded experimental possibilities. I would also note that conversations, conferences, lectures and texts have played a crucial role in my practice as an artist. Not content to work on projects that are continuations of predetermined genres, I instead look towards the biological realm and its sciences for ideas concerning alternative art-making possibilities. This notion is supported by the fact that this is, in numerous ways, a golden phase for the biological sciences and some would even say we live in a Biological Age. Somewhat oblique to the discourses operating within museum culture, biennials and art fairs, and art practice in general, my investigations remain unhindered. If art making is a data bank encompassing all other data banks as history has shown, then of course there is no arguing this point about relevance or content.[3]

Embedded in past and present biological ruminations and theories are a myriad number of topics reflecting the social, political and economic conditions of our globalized world. Issues concerning gender and reproductive rights, illicit and consensual body-part farming, food alteration and adulteration, xenotransplantation, life extensions and enhancements and the patenting and licensing of gene sequencing are some of the matters pervasive to these explorations. Allied fields in design and architecture have also brought forward methods by which microorganisms are being employed in building materials and even textiles.[4]

2 The Bio Art Laboratory at the BFA Fine Arts Department of the School of Visual Arts was originally named The Nature and Technology Lab (NAT Lab). Both names are in operation concerning the space, which incorporates biological investigation and its interface with technology.

3 This essay, available as part of the Appendix of this volume (p. 215), was previously published in "Viruses and Pearls: The Materialization of Culture." *N.A.P. text(s)* 1, no. 2 (1995): 14-15.

4 For examples of sustainable design see William Myers, *Bio Design: Nature, Science, Creativity* (New York: Museum of Modern Art, 2012).

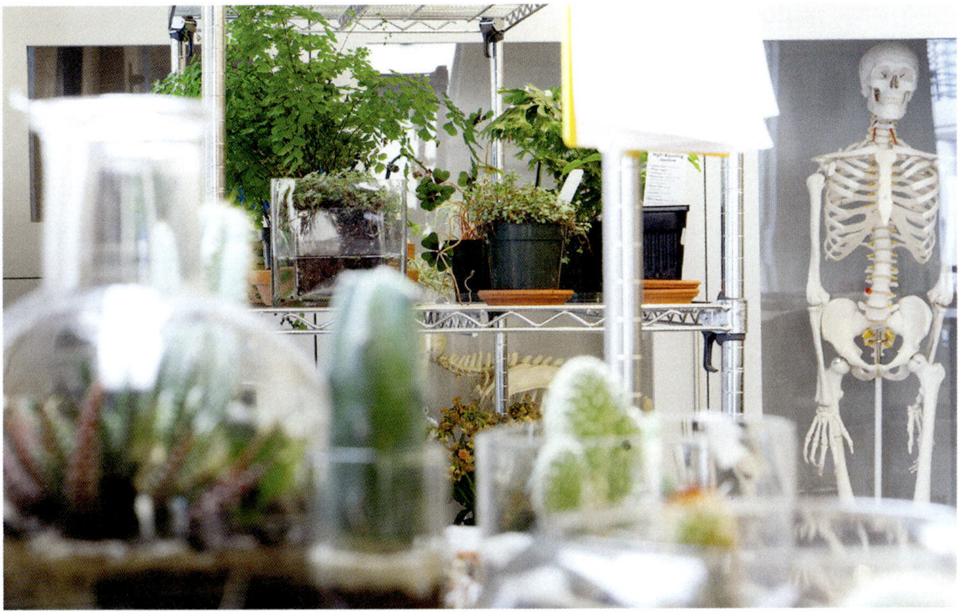

Figure 9. Botanical specimens and a full-figure anatomical skeleton at the School of Visual Arts' Bio Art Lab, BFA Fine Arts Department, New York City, 2012. Photograph by Raul Valverde.

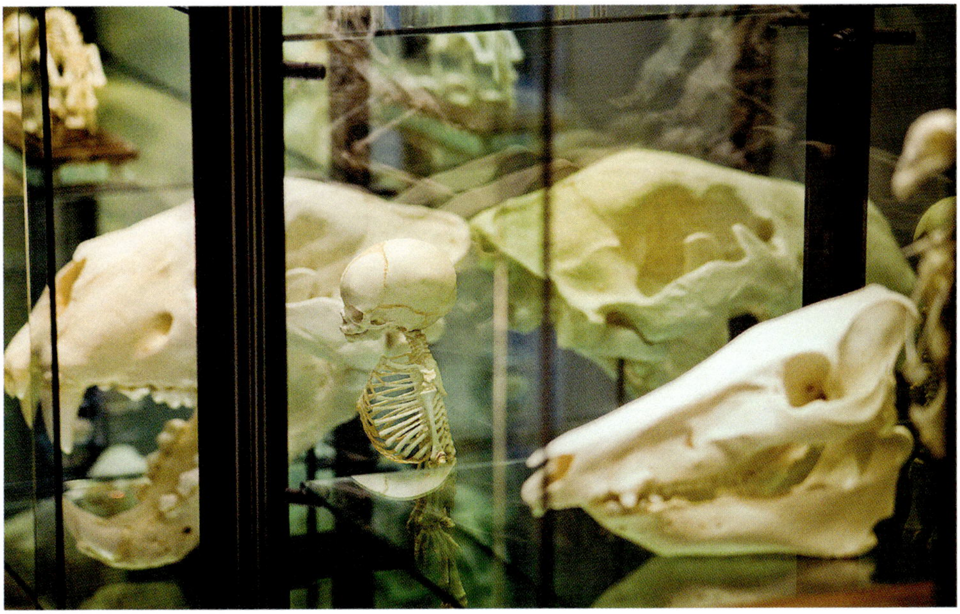

Figure 10. Skeleton collection for use in comparative anatomy drawing classes at the School of Visual Arts' Bio Art Lab, 2012. Photograph by Raul Valverde.

From Apocalypse to Analogy

If circumstance is the great leveler, I have been ready and able to move within its pride. These investigations continue at the present time, bringing me into fresh domains of thought and presence. My experiences, not circumscribed in this volume, include several extreme sites. An example is my visit to Auschwitz and Birkenau, where the stench of death boondoggles the mind. Although such foulness is not readily available to the senses, since the death camp "bunkers" have been refashioned, the grass has been manicured, and healthy trees and shrubs have been planted. It is with this erasure of death that it is even more evident that genuinely evil acts have unfolded here.

The infamous iron sign "ARBEIT MACHT FREI" translated as "work makes you free" placed at the entrance of the camp, ironically, is a replica. The original, stolen in 2009, was recovered and placed in the Auschwitz-Birkenau State Museum. Walking through the open gate gives one pause. Memories of wartime photographs and films sink into one's entire body, as if one is experiencing what the late poet Paul Celan called a land of "black milk."

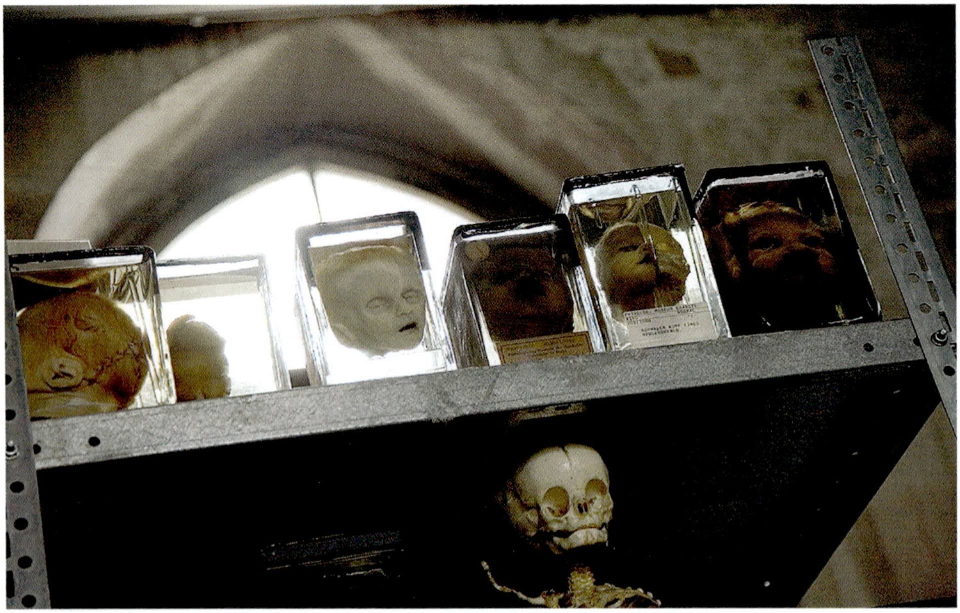

Figure 11. Suzanne Anker: *The Glass Veil (Shelley's Dream)*, 2009.
Inkjet print on sintra, 8.5 x 11 in (21.6 x 28 cm).

We are encouraged to remember Primo Levi's poem in his text, *If This Is a Man*[5]:

You who live safe
In your warm houses,
You who find, returning in the evening,
Hot food and friendly faces:
    Consider if this is a man
    Who works in the mud,
    Who does not know peace,
    Who fights for a scrap of bread,
    Who dies because of a yes or a no.
    Consider if this is a woman
    Without hair and without name,
    With no more strength to remember,
    Her eyes empty and her womb cold
    Like a frog in winter.
Meditate that this came about:
I commend these words to you.
Carve them in your hearts
At home, in the street,
Going to bed, rising;
Repeat them to your children.
    Or may your house fall apart,
    May illness impede you,
    May your children turn their faces from you

Can the solemnity of a death camp be converted into a commodity-driven theme park? Upon arrival visitors are given a colored sticker–yellow, purple, blue, green, red, etc. to attach to their clothing so that they become part of a group. How insensitive can such a gesture be? Were not the prisoners of the camps forced to wear such identifying insignias? Is color-coding appropriate in this case? As subject matter for artworks, at this point, I concede that my own sensibilities cannot engage this frame of historical time. I am numb in this regard in trying to comprehend the scale of such inhumanity and evil. I don't agree with philosopher Hannah Arendt's controversial supposition that "the banality of evil is the work of small obedient men."[6] There is nothing banal about evil and human responsibility.

---

5 Primo Levi, *If This Is a Man* (New York: Orion Press, 1959).

6 Hannah Arendt, *Eichmann in Jerusalem: A Report on the Banality of Evil* (New York: Penguin Books, 2006).

There is no way to rationalize enormously vicious crimes or even attribute their presence to lack of judgment.

While at the camps, however, I picked up some weeds and flowers, leaves and grass that have within them the genetic memory of both atrocity and survival. If trees could speak what would they say of their first hand experience as witnesses to such unforgiving heinousness and staggering disquietude? Perhaps one day I will be able to create a project concerning the horror and monstrousness of such actions. But what particularly struck me was the camp's geographical proximity to Krakow, a jewel of a city in Poland seemingly untarnished by the war. Additionally, on my short ride to Auschwitz from Krakow many private homes with residential occupants persist, forcing me to question how one can live comfortably in the presence of the residue of such malevolence? How was it unknown as to what was unfolding?

On a less sobering note is my excursion to Woods Hole, in Massachusetts, home to the Oceanographic Institution and the Marine Biological Laboratory (MBL)[7]. Surrounded by water and glimmering light, set in an idyllic cove, it is common to watch Nobel Prize recipients meander through the walkways in an ordinary manner. In this environment, I had the opportunity to work with marine biologist and neuroscientist, Joseph DeGiorgis. Here cold-water coral, jellyfish, plankton et al are studied as model organisms that can aid in extending human life and combat disease. It is here where research scientists speculate on the mechanisms of just how "life" works. The Oceanographic Institution, well known in popular culture, boasts of its pioneering scientist, Robert Ballard, who led a team of explorers to locate the Titanic in 1985. *The New York Times* noted that "ten millionaires were aboard and the safe storage room was filled with valuables, including diamonds valued at $7 million in 1912."[8] Diamonds and ice are a strange combination of affluence and disaster. They continue to attract humans – sometimes on a crusade for freedom and on other occasions stimulated by the seduction of revelation – to uncertainty and risk. Ballard and his team, however were on another mission, an undercover expedition funded by the United States Navy in search of two sunken American nuclear submarines, in which the sub-rosa "cover story" was the search for the Titanic.[9]

More pertinent to my work is the institute's encounter with hydrothermal vents in which a vast range of life forms can survive in the absence of light. Enabled with a method of food synthesis akin to photosynthesis, yet alternately

7 For more info about the Woods Hole Oceanographic Institution visit http://www.whoi.edu.

8 William Broad, "Wreckage of Titanic Reported Discovered 12,000 Feet Down," *The New York Times*, September 3, 1985.

9 Kit Eaton, "Hunt for Titanic Was Cover for Secret Sunken Nuke Sub Dives," *Gizmodo*, May 26, 2008.

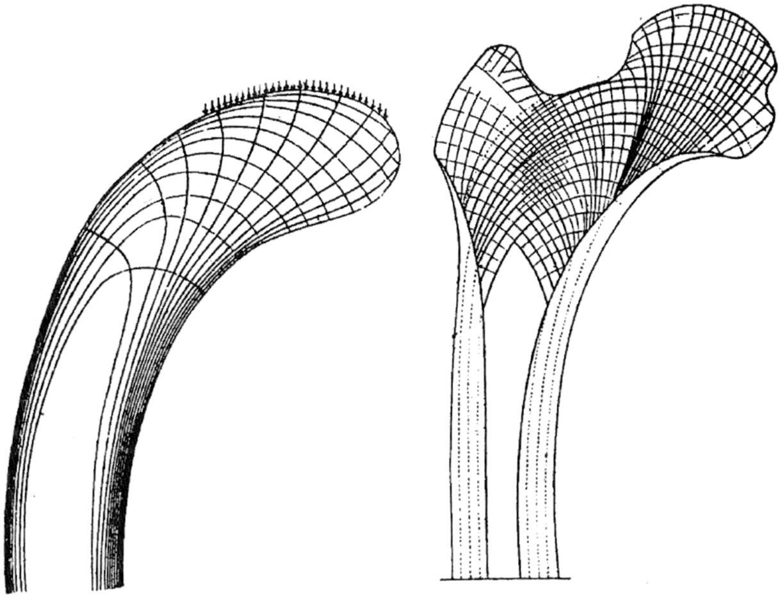

Figure 12. Crane-head and femur. After Culmann and J. Wolff. Illustration from D'Arcy Wentworth Thompson's text *On Growth and Form* (Cambridge: Cambridge University Press, 1968), 233.

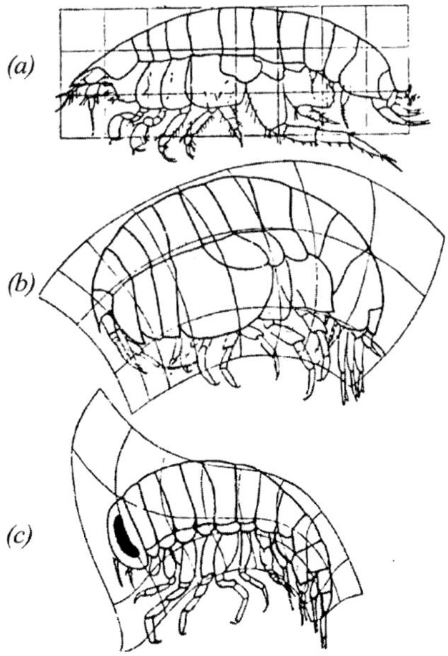

Figure 13. (a) *Harpinia plumosa* Kr.; (b) *Stegocephalus inflatus* Kr.; (c) *Hyperia galba.* Illustration from D'Arcy Wentworth Thompson's text *On Growth and Form* (Cambridge: Cambridge University Press, 1968), 295.

special, these creatures are able to employ "terrestrial energy" in which chemolithoautotrophic bacteria assume the role of green plants."[10]My work illustrated in Dialogue III of this volume, *Origins and Futures* addresses a theory of the origin of life referring to primitive RNA. This primordial molecule, according to A.G. Cairns-Smith's hypothesis, captured the crystalline structure of minerals and thus learned to replicate copies of itself. These unique manifestations attest to the ways in which nature continually stupefies us with expedient methods of creation. What we assume to be universally factual is, of course, only valid on a temporary basis. Exposing new problematics is part of the variegated practices embedded in the disciplines of research science and the visual arts. Such exponential variation is of course in sync with Darwin's "tangled bank" of all interrelated living forms.

My visit to Dundee, Scotland, took me to the D'Arcy Thompson Zoology Museum, located at the University of Dundee. It is here where the eminent biologist D'Arcy Thompson was appointed Chair of the Biology Department before taking up residence at St. Andrews. The museum houses the remnants of his collections such as animal skeletons, anatomical models, as well as biological charts and diagrams. His extraordinary work accounts for exceptionally great strides in the mathematical roots of form. His seminal text *On Growth and Form* has had a reverberating influence on many artists, particularly the American Abstract Expressionists who looked towards nature as a way to remake the world after World War II.

The significance of D'Arcy Thompson for my work is evident in my sculptures that employ rapid prototype technologies. Because such 3D software programs have the ability to turn numbers into form–and form into numbers–the mathematical calculations are instant. In the days of Thompson, complex equations were required to decipher physical causation and efficiency of forms (figs. 12-13). Linear maps, referred to as wire frames, are mathematically-derived representations calculated by three-dimensional modeling programs. Such images parallel Thompson's work, which serve as a reference to my series of prints titled *Spiral Maze* (2014) (figs. 14-16). In his own words, Thompson was concerned with forms that could be imagined. In his text he states: "Our own study of organic form, which we call by Goethe's name of Morphology, is but a portion of that wider Science of Form which deals with the forms assumed by matter under all aspects and conditions, and, in a still wider sense, with forms which are theoretically imaginable."The pertinence of this statement in the 21st century, is quite significant since with current software programs it is possible to construct a model,

10 Jannasch Holger, "Microbial Sulfur Oxidation and Deep-Sea Hydrothermal Vents," *Small is Powerful: Recollections of a Microbiologist and Oceanographer. Annual Review of Microbiology* 51 (1997): 25.

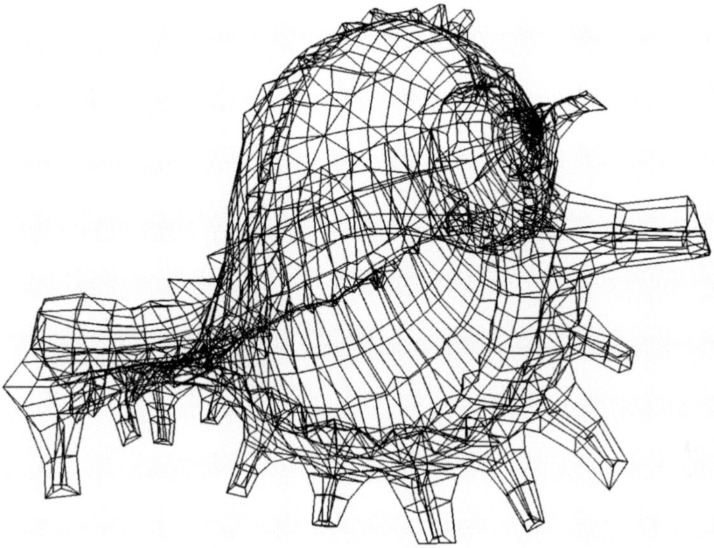

Figure 14. Suzanne Anker: *Spiral Maze 1*, 2014. Computer-generated wireframe study for silk-screen and inkjet print. Collaboration with Dr. Paul Harrison, Visual Research Center, Duncan of Jordanstone College of Art and Design, University of Dundee, Scotland.

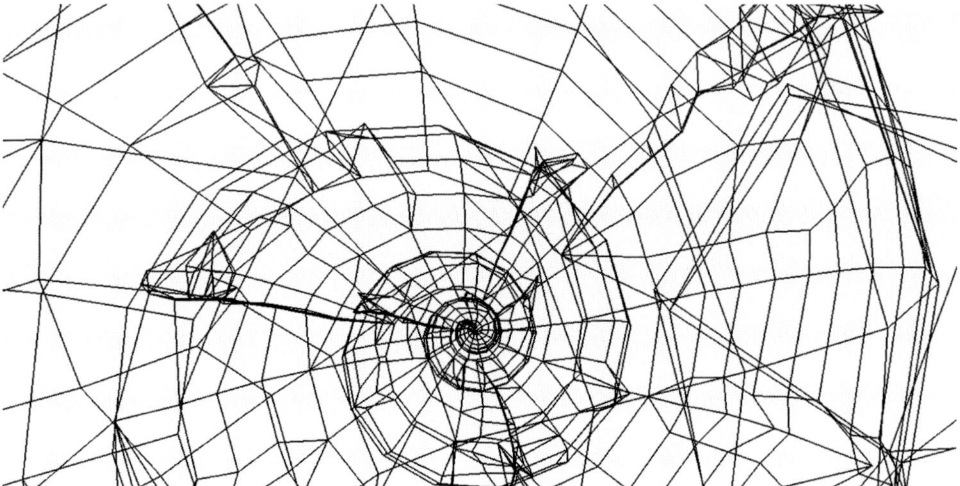

Figure 15. Suzanne Anker: *Spiral Maze 2*, 2014. Computer-generated wireframe study for silk-screen and inkjet print. Collaboration with Dr. Paul Harrison.

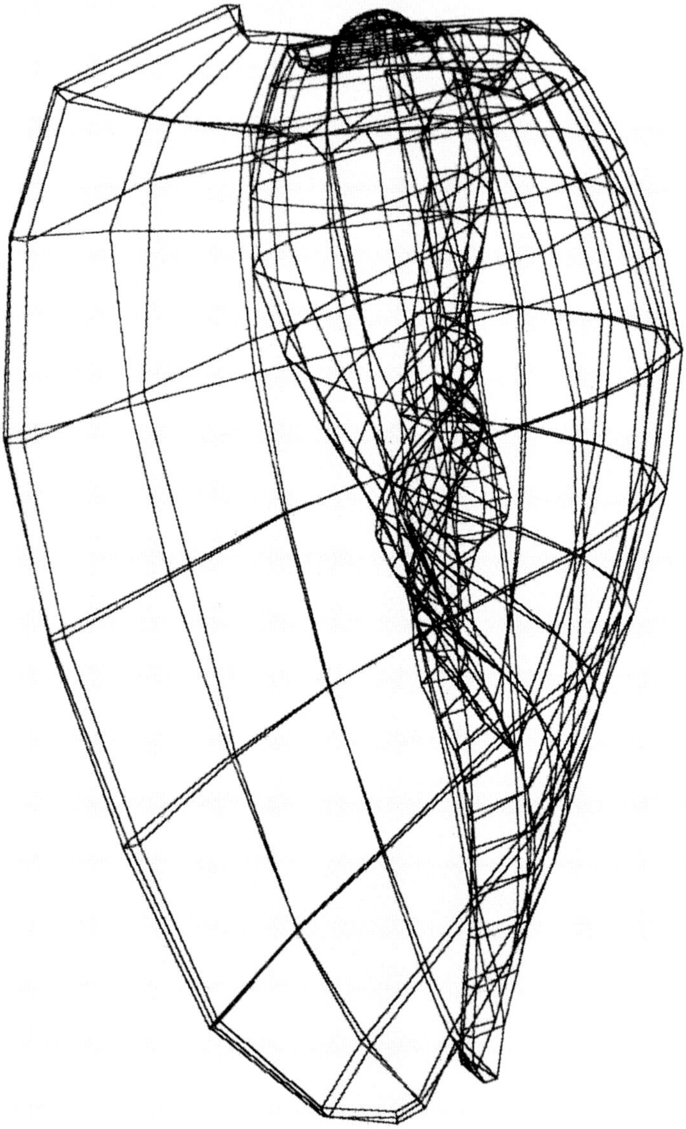

Figure 16. Suzanne Anker: *Spiral Maze 3*, 2014. Computer-generated wireframe study for silk-screen and inkjet print. Collaboration with Dr. Paul Harrison.

which on a larger scale cannot be built. Whereas code can combine without the intrusion of matter, matter is circumspect to the variables of space and its forces.

Another recent excursion in June 2014, brought me to the University of Cambridge in the United Kingdom as part of an expert meeting on *In Vitro Fertilization* (IVF) and reproductive technologies. Cambridge is the site of the first "test tube baby," Louise Brown, who came into existence in 1976. Robert Edwards and his team of researchers, which included Sir Richard Gardner and Bob Moor, were extremely interested in the underlying causes of genetic inheritance and looked towards in vitro methods of culturing blastocysts in an attempt to understand Down, Klinefelter and Turner syndromes. Such techniques required fertilization to occur outside the womb for later transplantation. In this procedure, human eggs and sperm are combined in a Petri dish to form a zygote. The resultant blastocyst is coaxed to divide and divide again until the correct number of cells are present.[11] This laboratory externalization of what was once a private affair of sexual reproduction takes a scientific turn, in which sexual contact is absent, heralding in an ongoing asexual revolution.

Originally met with skepticism, fear and awe, these techniques extend today into a multi-billion dollar enterprise. Procedures relating to the freezing and thawing of embryos, retrieval of sperm and acquisition of eggs, have expanded the availability of these techniques. What health ramifications and social side effects become part of such familial landscapes as new industries of surrogacy and cryo-embryology spawn new corporate undertakings? Writing this text in June of 2014, I glance at the cover of the magazine section of the *New York Times*, only to find the cover image and subsequent article is about three-parent IVF treatments. This is a technology that requires a third parent's cytoplasm, which is injected into the birth mother's egg. Cytoplasm carries mitochondrial DNA, a separate genome consisting of thirty-seven chromosomes, which passes from mother to daughter and thereon afterwards. At this stage of development, this procedure called cytoplasmic transfer is a radical biological technique which also calls into question the issue of kinship, since it is a method that crosses the germ-line of inheritance.[12]

11 Gina Kolata, "Robert G. Edwards Dies at 87: Changed Rules of Conception With First Test Tube Baby," *The New York Times*, April 10, 2013.

12 Kim Tingley, "The Brave New World of Three-Parent IVF." *The New York Times*, June 27, 2014, MM26.

Transforming Life

If we look at the possibilities of an expanded notion of aesthetics, criss-crossing myriad disciplines, the practice of art is a revitalizing agent with transforming capabilities. As we learn from the biological sciences and geographical flux, borders are temporary injunctions playing out current access to power relations, such is true in the art world itself. Although many discourses are seemingly fixed, we can still ponder notions of individual excellence or grace, which breach the rules of discontented status quos. Of course, such independence comes at a price, but what else is more commanding?

Throughout art history and visual culture, numerous tales of "messing with nature" are stern warnings in advance of mankind's hubris and ultimate destruction. Whether we invoke Mary Shelley's classic *Frankenstein; The Modern Prometheus* or Aldous Huxley's *Brave New World* or Margaret Atwood's trilogy of *Oryx and Crake*, each story embodies a future where nature's revenge is fiercely expressed. However daunting these warnings remain, they do not alter man's predilection for acquiring and re-attributing knowledge.

In this time of uncertainty and geopolitical reconfiguration, what intellectual plateaus and genus of aesthetic output reverberate with the times? As concepts of the avant-garde continue to wither away under the protuberances of heavy-loaded discourse, how can such forces of consternation and dissolution be held at bay? Are we doomed to endorse mass culture's reigning paradigm of "playground aesthetics"? What role does art assume beyond its international exchange value?

In the pursuit of innovation, many artists, designers, filmmakers, writers and architects look towards emerging fields of speculative design in which ideas of open-ended invention predominate. Referring to their work as discoverable solutions, Anthony Dunne and Fiona Raby discuss an approach for "achieving desirable futures" in their text, *Speculative Everything: Design, Fiction and Social Dreaming*. They are part of a generation of innovators, who explore numerous hypothetical and unorthodox approaches. For example, DIY Biology is an international movement of bio hackers who repurpose defunct laboratory equipment, give classes in open source labs, and rent laboratory space to community participants. These actions circumvent conventional institutional protocol and regulations. BioCurious, in San Francisco, California and Genspace in Brooklyn, New York, are not-for-profit community bio laboratory spaces of this order. Visionary architecture and urban planning in the work of Mitchell Joachim of Terreform ONE looks towards population eruption in global terms, projecting hot spots of population growth and consumer contamination. Other practitioners include Shiho Fukuhara and Georg Tremmel who breed genetically altered flowers in reverse so as to attain the plant's original color and form. Lisa Ma, working with laborers in China, creates improved working conditions for migrant "joystick factory workers."[13] In this project, the employees are able to farm their own food, bringing them closer to what they consider to be meaningful work. Vik Muniz's powerful film *Waste Land*, offers a glimpse into the world of "garbage pickers" in Brazil where they sort through trash to garner metal and other fungible goods. Such "pickings" are exchanged for currency as a way to support themselves and their families.

Enigmatic questions are no surprise to any discipline, or for that matter, to ordinary research or imaginative impressions. As the ways and means to transform and alter life begin their journey from a Petri dish to a living organism, how are we to embrace these novel methods and forms? As we mix and match parts of genetic sequences, combining them with phylogenetic others, what new organisms can be fabricated? How will these organisms be embedded into the "natural" world and what status will be given to them?

There is much discussion about science in this volume, and perhaps not enough about art. However, the science presented here is inexorably linked to art in that the visuals presented draw their inspiration from the biological sciences, but they remain as represented – works of art. Bio Art, a yet-to-be sorted out category, may be a critical reference for extrapolating such intersections. It is understood that science always has a second life: first as material discovery or application and secondly as cultural indicator. Currency, not in the monetary sense, but in the arena of current events, creates for art practice an ever-expanding archive of postulates from which to draw. As with all sign systems, cultural expression is a litmus test connected to a cultural imaginary which functions as a barometer, measuring a society's reflection upon itself.

---

13 For more information about the *Farmification* project by Lisa Ma, visit http://fringejoyride.com/category/joystick-factory.

References

Anker, Suzanne. "Viruses and Pearls: The Materialization of Culture." *N.A.P. text(s). The Arts Program. Kutztown, PA* 1, no. 2: 14-15.

Arendt, Hannah. *Eichmann in Jerusalem: A Report on the Banality of Evil*. New York, N.Y., U.S.A.: Penguin Books, 2006.

Atwood, Margaret. *Oryx and Crake: A Novel*. New York: Nan A. Talese, 2003.

Broad, William. "Wreckage of Titanic Reported Discovered 12,000 Feet Down." *The New York Times*, September 3, 1985: C6.

Cairns-Smith, A. G. *Seven Clues to the Origin of Life A Scientific Detective Story*. Cambridge [England]: Cambridge University Press, 1990.

Dunne, Anthony, and Fiona Raby. *Speculative Everything: Design, Fiction, and Social Dreaming*. Cambridge (Mass.): MIT Press, 2013.

Eaton, Kit. "Hunt for Titanic Was Cover for Secret Sunken Nuke Sub Dives." Gizmodo (blog). May 26, 2008. http://gizmodo.com/393211/hunt-for-titanic-was-cover-for-secret-sunken-nuke-sub-dives.

Felstiner, John. *Paul Celan: Poet, Survivor, Jew*. New Haven: Yale University Press, 1995.

Huxley, Aldous. *Brave New World*. New York: Harper & Bros, 1946.

Jannasch, Holger. "Microbial Sulfur Oxidation and Deep-Sea Hydrothermal Vents." *Small is Powerful: Recollections of a Microbiologist and Oceanographer. Annual Review of Microbiology* 51 (1997): 25.

Kolata, Gina. "Robert G. Edwards Dies at 87: Changed Rules of Conception With First Test Tube Baby." *The New York Times*, April 10, 2013.

Kollwitz, Käthe, and Hans Kollwitz. *The Diary and Letters of Kaethe Kollwitz*. Evanston, Ill: Northwestern University Press, 1988.

Levi, Primo. *If This Is a Man*. New York: Orion Press, 1959.

Myers, William. *Bio Design: Nature, Science, Creativity*. New York: Museum of Modern Art, 2012.

Thompson, D'Arcy Wentworth. *On Growth and Form*, 12th ed. Cambridge: Cambridge University Press, 1968.

Tingley, Kim. "The Brave New World of Three-Parent IVF." *The New York Times*, June 27, 2014.

Waste Land. Directed by Lucy Walker. 2010. UK, Brasil Film.

List of Illustrations

Fig. 9: Botanical specimens and full-figure anatomical skeleton at the School of Visual Arts' Bio Art Lab, BFA Fine Arts Department, New York City, 2012. Photograph by Raul Valverde.

Fig. 10: Skeleton collection for use in comparative anatomy drawing classes at the School of Visual Arts' Bio Art Lab, BFA Fine Arts Department, New York City, 2012. Photograph by Raul Valverde.

Fig. 11: Suzanne Anker: *The Glass Veil (Shelley's Dream)*, 2009. Inkjet print on sintra, 8.5 x 11 in (21.6 x 28 cm).

Fig. 12. Illustration from D'Arcy Wentworth Thompson's text *On Growth and Form* (Cambridge: Cambridge University Press, 1968), 233.

Fig. 13. Illustration from D'Arcy Wentworth Thompson's text *On Growth and Form* (Cambridge: Cambridge University Press, 1968), 295.

Fig. 14: Suzanne Anker: *Spiral Maze 1*, 2014. Computer-generated wireframe study for silkscreen and inkjet print on archival paper, 22 x 30 in (76 x 56 cm). Collaboration with Dr. Paul Harrison, Visual Research Center, Duncan of Jordanstone College of Art and Design, University of Dundee, Scotland.

Fig. 15: Suzanne Anker: *Spiral Maze 2*, 2014. Computer-generated wireframe study for silkscreen and inkjet print on archival paper, 22 x 30 in (76 x 56 cm). Collaboration with Dr. Paul Harrison, Visual Research Center, Duncan of Jordanstone College of Art and Design, University of Dundee, Scotland.

Fig. 16: Suzanne Anker: *Spiral Maze 3*, 2014. Computer-generated wireframe study for silkscreen and inkjet print on archival paper, 22 x 30 in (76 x 56 cm). Collaboration with Dr. Paul Harrison, Visual Research Center, Duncan of Jordanstone College of Art and Design, University of Dundee, Scotland.

Through the Looking Glass: Encounters with Suzanne Anker's Wonderlands

SABINE FLACH

I. Making is Thinking – Art as Knowledge

> The people nowadays believe that the scientists are there to teach them, and the poets, musicians and artists, etc. to please them. *That the latter might have something to teach* is not something they consider.[1]

This remark is found in one of Ludwig Wittgenstein's notebooks. If, according to Wittgenstein, the arts teach us something, then they must manifest a form of knowledge. It is this knowledge, the knowledge that we find in art, which is the subject matter of what follows. I suggest here, first, that art possesses a specific, irreducible and characteristic domain of knowledge; hence my reflections focus on the particular and productive qualities of art itself. The second train of thought is the assumption that as soon as the knowledge of art is examined, the traditional distinction between theory and practice becomes redundant. As I argue, the two modalities of knowledge production are interlaced in the artwork as artwork – it is characteristic of art to govern production and result in the work itself.

With regard to the dialogic relation between art and science, I suggest a sharpening of focus regarding the distinctions, as opposed to problematic positions demanding the de-differentiation of the two fields. It is, however, not my aim to construct impenetrable boundaries, but rather to make productive use of the differences. And to do so with the aim of a collaborative relation of the fields in terms of complimentary questions and solutions. For there is little sense in simply defining away the methodological, epistemological and habitual differences between technology and the natural sciences on the one hand and the arts and humanities on the other.

The question of just how artistic knowledge becomes visible within this complex, and what its concrete function is, might be illuminated through a theoretical engagement attempting to consider art as a research discipline equal to the natural sciences, and marking intersections both in terms of historical contextualization and the methodological grounding of these attempts.

1 Ludwig Wittgenstein, *Vermischte Bemerkungen. Eine Auswahl aus dem Nachlass* (Frankfurt/ Main: Suhrkamp, 1994), 79. Unless otherwise stated, all translations of quotations are by Lisa Jeschke.

Hence Paul Valéry's reflections on art circle around the assumption that the division between art and science can only be maintained from a perspective of not taking account of the production process of an object and instead focusing exclusively on the end product.[2] His attention, by contrast, is not so much directed on results, but on the intersections of science and art, emphasizing moments of construction.[3] Such an approach, however, does not negate the differences of the two realms; rather, we observe a shift towards a field of subtle distinctions. Hence in his Leonardo essay, Valéry suggests that the realms differ only "après les variations, d'un fond commun, par ce qu'ils en conservent et ce qu'ils en négligent, en formant leurs langages et leurs symboles."[4] What remains common to both the arts and the sciences is the '*combinatorics*' of elements. The differential lies in the modalities of sorting and separating and in the aim and function, that is, the framework upon which a statement depends. And this is to be reconsidered for each particular case.

Hence it is necessary to acknowledge processes of distinction as well as blending different forms of knowledge, moments of differentiation as well as of intersection and contact–the assemblage of hybrid knowledge formations circulating between the cultures. It is not the obvious relations that are being addressed here, but those faculties of art which provide the transdisciplinarity in the first place.

Against what appears to be the ahistoricity of current discussions regarding artistic knowledge and research, we find ourselves within a paragone that has been running for a long time: the arts and sciences have always been competitive in terms of maintaining their ground in relation to what we know, where that knowledge occurs and how it might be described. One of the outstanding examples is the artistic research conducted by the classical avant-gardes. The conception of artist and artwork, developed during this period, established a markedly different understanding of artistic activity.

Kasimir Malevich,[5] for instance, was interested in understanding art as a science in order to develop new pedagogic practices and to diffuse these, at a

2 What is interesting to Valéry, however, is not the work but the liminal space resulting from the collision of two different realms: "J'ai combiné les termes suivantes, peinture, architecture, mathématique, mécanique, physique et mécanismes (...)," he notes after finishing his Introduction à la méthode de Léonard de Vinci. It is the development of the artwork which he describes as its "embryo state" (sic!) which forms the nucleus of Valéry's theoretical reflection, for: "In this state, the difference between scientist and artist dissolves. At this stage, there is nothing but the play of excitement, of attention, of coincidence and of mental states."

3 Paul Valéry, *Oeuvres*, vol. 1 (Paris: Gallimard, 1990), 22.

4 Ibid., 157.

5 He was invested in the relation between art and knowledge from 1918 onwards, during his occupation at the Moscow Free State Art Studios (SVOMAS), which was renamed in 1920 as Vkhutemas (Higher Art and Technical Studios). Further, around 1920 the group UNOVIS–The Champions of the New Art–was assembled around Malevich.

later stage, into further systems of knowledge;[6] to quote Malevich, "to oppose two methods of taste in terms of 'like–dislike' [as] a scientific approach (doing away with) the previous conception of the painter and replacing the painter with the scientist".[7] It is along these lines that demands made upon the artist and ideas respecting artistic activity were to change. Because of their research, their knowledge, and their methodologies, artists advanced to become directors of departments at various institutes conducting research which in a more conservative climate would only have been granted to scientists and supporting scholars.

Apropos to the premise of an exhaustive investigation of perception, for instance, Mikhail Matyushin conducted, in his laboratory, experiments and research regarding kinaesthetic and synaesthetic vision. The scurrility of his ideas aside, Matyushin was against sensualist kinds of theories of perception. According to Matyushin, it is the modal variety of the senses which forms a subject's constitutive qualities.[8]

Wassily Kandinsky – an artist, not a scientist – was among the most advanced thinkers and representatives of artistic knowledge. At the Bauhaus he ran a 'scientific' research department of psycho-physics and its problems. He ceaselessly argued for the competency of art and for overcoming the separation between the arts and sciences. His plea against specialization is directed towards the not fully severed connective lines between the arts and the sciences – in spite of the dominance of positivism and the analytical sciences. But Kandinsky did not argue for a crude merging – rather for a focus on traces uniting the two areas, as well as on phenomena of convergence, made possible perhaps precisely as a result of specialization processes. Hence the developments of the nineteenth century might be given a positive turn so as to complement them and make use of them.[9] Kandinsky posited artistic epistemological functions as absolute, and developed from them the idea of a synthetic method. Synthesis – in contrast to analysis – was from now on to dominate progressive sciences – among them, art.[10]

6 Also see: Selim Khan-Magomedov, *Vhutemas*: Moscou 1920-1930, vol. 2 (Paris: Editions du Regard, 1990).

7 Sabine Flach, *Körper-Szenarien: Zum Verhältnis von Körper und Bild in Videoinstallationen* (Munich: Wilhelm Fink, 2003).

8 Matyushin was able to show that the senses and the body always already constitute a synergic system.

9 The arts – and artists – occupy an outstanding position in Kandinsky's ensemble, not only in the practical, but also in the theoretical work which considers the rejection of theory produced by artists as a position belonging to the past; according to Kandinsky, "most writing on art is produced by people who are not artists: thus all the wrong concepts and judgements."

10 Wassily Kandinsky, "Die Grundelemente der Form." In *Essays über Kunst und Künstler*, ed. by Wassily Kandinsky et al. (Bern: Benteli, 1963), 71.

II. "We can know more than we can tell"

Martin Heidegger recognized as paradoxical the privileging of language in the explication of scientific and artistic phenomena and events: "Speaking of language, we remain entangled in continually insufficient speech. Such an entanglement closes us off from that which is to make itself known to thought." The philosopher considered as the only possibility of escaping verbalization to "take note of that which is specific to the track of knowledge, that is, to look around the region where thinking is situated."[11]

What is meant by looking around the region where thinking is situated? How can this "region," a spatial configuration, be recognized, and how can artistic thought be recognized within it? How can a form of knowledge that evades exclusive focus on language be produced, found and experienced? What is the theoretical space that needs to be constructed in order for this knowledge to be able to reveal itself?

"We can know more than we can tell," the philosopher Michael Polanyi states in his 1966 publication *The Tacit Dimension*, about the difficulty of grasping knowledge. Acquiring knowledge is not a simple thing: in Meno's paradox, Plato writes that "it is not possible for man to search, neither that which he knows nor that which he does not know. For he will not search for that which he knows, given that he knows it, and whoever is capable need not look further, nor for that which he does not know; for he does not know what to look for."[12]

Polanyi's suggestion, which I will initially follow here, is to introduce the concept of "tacit knowledge"–an implied kind of knowledge which is always already understood as part of knowledge in that it clarifies what the aim of epistemological inquiry might be in the first place, and what one wants to know. One of the implications for Polanyi is that "the process of formalizing all knowledge to the exclusion of tacit knowledge is self-defeating."[13]

Polanyi develops "tacit knowledge" in close proximity to Gestalt theory, based on the assumption that knowledge contains elements which escape formalization and an exact verbalization. In this respect, Polanyi remarks: "The structure of Gestalt is then recast into a logic of tacit thought, and this changes the range and perspective of the whole subject. The highest forms of integration loom largest now. These are manifested in the tacit power of scientific and *artistic* genius. The art of expert diagnosticians may be listed next, as a somewhat impoverished form of discovery, and we may put in the same class the performance of skills,

11 Martin Heidegger, *Unterwegs zur Sprache* (Stuttgart: Klett-Cotta, 2007), 179.

12 Plato. *Meno* (Stuttgart: Reclam, 2010), 80d-e.

13 Michael Polanyi, *The Tacit Dimension* (Chicago: University of Chicago Press, 2009), xi.

whether artistic (...) or technical. We have here examples of *knowing*, both of a more intellectual and more practical kind, both the 'wissen' and 'können' of the Germans or the 'knowing what' and 'knowing how' (...). Both of these *aspects of knowing have a similar structure and neither is ever present without the other.* (...) True knowledge lies in our ability to use it."[14]

Polanyi's fundamental conviction concerning the impossibility of separating knowledge, experience, perception, etc. from a personalization of knowledge is what interests me in terms of his conception of tacit knowledge, as well as its phenomenological and ontological aspects. Nevertheless, as I suggest, it is necessary to develop his considerations further; for even if his approach of acknowledging that art contains an implied form of knowledge seems useful, such a positioning remains bound to a conventional frame of reference which cannot clarify how exactly knowledge that is implicit may become explicit.

In what follows, these reflections are further explicated in relation to the work of American artist Suzanne Anker. Her works might be understood as a pars pro toto for artistic research in the best possible sense of transdisciplinarity. Her work has always positioned itself at the intersection points of various knowledge concepts, knowledge disciplines, media and techniques. What is produced in her research activity is the visualization of complex structures of knowledge, and the area within which this research is situated is, determinately: art. I will focus on two of the artist's work complexes which occupy meaning in differing ways, and with processes by which an image is perceived.

III. Ars Quaerendi–The Art of Asking Questions

"(I present) zones of ambiguity in which images recall an unimaginable presence. What does it feel like for a viewer to be confronted by a brain or a fetus floating in fluids on display? How does one address personhood with regard to these images? Dead, but yet still animated by reflected light. Akin to looking into an aquarium, viewers are confronted with the anthropomorphic nature of these fragments cum beings. Although these 'cuttings' remain dead, they still perform a function in the living world"[15]–this is how Suzanne Anker describes the project The Glass Veil which we developed together between 2007 and 2009 and which was exhibited in a solo show in Berlin in 2009.

14 Ibid., 7 and 17. Emphases S. Flach.

15 Suzanne Anker and Sabine Flach. "The Glass Veil." In *Habitas in Habitas: Emotion and Motion*, ed. Daniel Margulies et al. (Berlin: Peter Lang, 2010), 146.

The installation *The Glass Veil* is the result of a close collaboration with Thomas Schnalke, the museum's director, and staff members of the Medizinhistorisches Museum der Charité. This collaboration involved conversations as well as observations of work processes conducted by the doctors at the Charité and by the curators of the museum's preparation halls. Anker's installation, in part, interrogates procedures and technologies of scientific visualization in various media. In short: the aim was to demonstrate how concepts of knowledge influence our perception of environments and of objects positioned in these environments.

But how might the skill of asking questions succeed so as to be able to research, via artistic means, the complexity of influences and make them available in an artistic compendium of knowledge? How is it possible to integrate an artistic form of knowledge that shows how, why and through what channels we produce, remember, acquire, change and pass on our knowledge through works of art?

Mnemosyne Atlas is the name Aby Warburg gave to what is probably the most famous compendium of the modes of operation of visual composition and their passage through cultural history. Warburg replaces iconography with art history as an archive of images. The logic of the image arrangement is not elaborated verbally; there is no textual element to explain the juxtaposition, the form of thought.[16] *Mnemosyne* – that is, the art of memory – questions how visual codes are produced, transformed and changed, while retaining their meaning as they are passed on. Considering himself not an art historian but a "historian of images" (*Bildgeschichtler*), Warburg was invested in "defining images [...] in the broadest sense and their effects as a 'laboratory of image history in terms of cultural studies'. Non-hierarchical fields of images are employed for the exploration of the *migration* of image motifs: through history, and *askew* in relation to disciplinary positions. It was Warburg's aim to locate an image motif in paintings, objects, popular culture, design, etc. so as to achieve 'the science of visual composition'."[17] Such a methodology centrally involves processes of memory: the memory of and about images, of their significance and application. What is crucial is to explore the knowledge within images as such, and their ability to actively *form* knowledge.

16 In his publication *Politische Landschaft. Zur Kunstgeschichte der Natur*, Hamburg-based art historian Martin Warnke attempts to take up the atlas' conventions of representation. In order to do so, Warnke divides each chapter into two parts, one of which presents its argument visually, the other one of which does so verbally. "In order to emphasize the perception I am interested in, I have left the textual and the image-based sections autonomous from one another: they are related only through a keyword but constitute separate statements." Martin Warnke, *Politische Landschaft. Zur Kunstgeschichte der Natur* (Munich: Hanser, 1992), 10.

17 Ibid.

This is also fundamental for Suzanne Anker. *The Glass Veil* involves not only those objects, instruments and histological specimens which formed part of the collection's holdings, but also some hidden aspects; such as sites and objects of which the visual preparation no longer accords with current standard practice. Hence her work does not merely reproduce that which has already been shown. Rather, her approach to objects exposes *ways of seeing*– in the double meaning of seeing: as a mode of seeing (perceiving as well as being supposed to see something) and as a positioning in terms of how seeing safeguards what is supposed and permitted to be seen. As a result, these works are much more than a mere confirmation of the fact that everything natural is also marked by the artificial. They disclose information with regard to the rules of composition and consequently with regard to what is intended as knowledge as part of the process of composition–in this case, medical objects and pathological specimens. What is being demonstrated is the dominance of a cultural, that is, a *socially mediated* aesthetic and its modes of recognizing and sanctioning. Suzanne Anker succeeds with such a demonstration *precisely by* reclaiming these images for art, wherein their cultural coding becomes apparent.

Where the aim is to examine the knowledge of art and its research aspects, it is crucial to focus on methodologies, techniques, processes and products–the manifest forms of *artistic theorization.* This implies a conceptualization of the image far beyond mere representation, a weaving together of "the world with figures of knowledge".[18] The image is then always a form of compression in which past and current impressions combine to form a figure of knowledge.[19] These processes involve divergent ways of engaging images and the different types and media of visual representation. And they unravel unaccounted for connections, that is, hidden or invisible complexities. To put it differently: these processes uncover zones of non-knowledge hidden within knowledge as blind spots and exclusions, spaces of negation and the unconscious, all of which form a correlation to knowledge, providing it with its contours and outline.

The following reflections will consequently be less concerned with the knowledge represented by images than with the production and structure of knowledge in the medium of images. These reflections will be concerned with the image as

18 W. J. T. Mitchell, *Picture Theory: Essays on Verbal and Visual Representation* (Chicago: University of Chicago Press, 1994).

19 Just as described by Walter Benjamin: "The image is that wherein that which has been forms a constellation with that which is now in a lightning-like instant." [Walter Benjamin *Das Passagenwerk*, vol. 1, ed. Rolf Tiedemann, (Frankfurt/Main: Suhrkamp, 1982), 576.] Cf. also Sigrid Weigel, "Bilder als Hauptakteure auf dem Schauplatz der Erkenntnis. Zur poiesis und episteme sprachlicher und visueller Bilder." In *Ästhetik – Erfahrung : Interventionen*, ed. Wlad Godzich et al. (Zürich: Springer, 2004).

an epistemological medium and model. Questions explicating how images generate meaning and uncover evidence employ inner reflections as an approach addressing forms of perception. Hence, I am especially interested in demonstrating that an image appears in a specific manner, enacting its own ontological presence which separates it from topical objects. Thus, images are processes which never repeat, but are engaged in rendering the visible.[20] What is it that renders visible the essence of an image – acting in a relation of difference vis-à-vis objects?

The Glass Veil, the title of Suzanne Anker's project, might provide a hint – pointing to transparency and indicating a shift of medium. A veil does not grant the possibility of looking *through* something, rather *into* something, directing mechanisms of seeing and perceiving while turning the observer into an agent, a spy or partner in terms of the attempt to locate the source of knowledge.[21] As Suzanne Anker works with given and found materials, her position as author can be described as *ex*-centric. In terms of a meaning of her images, their function is neither that of the absolute originator nor is she the final instance of signification. Suzanne Anker's work consists of the selection of materials, of the determination of the image excerpt and of the choice of specific procedures in terms of medium and technique. Such a working process entails subtle and yet definite and marked modifications. Artistic work in this case involves, on the one hand, an intervention in relation to that which has already been formulated[22], one's self-inscription into given images and experimentation with materials; and on the other hand, the presentation of that which already exists, the administration of techniques, a witnessing of events, and the preservation of traces which are concealed.

For example, we might say with regard to the image *The Hand Mirror* (see Dialogue I, fig. 19, p.74) that the preserved specimen is an object appearing like a painting. Anker's compositional technique is certainly not based on unambiguousness in the choice of media. Instead, the work draws our attention to how an object is perceived; the object appears precisely not as a preparation but re-

20 Gottfried Boehm, "Die Wiederkehr der Bilder." In *Was ist ein Bild?*, ed. Gottfried Boehm, (Munich: Wilhelm Fink, 2006), 33.

21 It is striking that in this respect, too, artistic production coalesces with Aby Warburg's propositions regarding a methodology of cultural theory. In his introduction of the *Mnemosyne Atlas*, Warburg grants special importance to the artistic person, writing: "We might consider the conscious distancing between self and the outside world as a foundational act of human civilization: when this gap turns into the substratum of artistic composition, the prerequisites towards making such a consciousness of distance a durable social function are fulfilled." Aby Warburg, Gertrud Bing, and Fritz Rougemont, *Gesammelte Schriften* (Leipzig: B.G. Teubner, 1932), 423.

22 Also see Stefan Germer, "Rückblick nach vorn." In *Jahresring 46. Germeriana Unveröffentlichte oder übersetzte Schriften von Stefan Germer zur zeitgenössischen und modernen Kunst*, ed. Julia Bernard (Cologne: DuMont, 1999), 92.

sembles a fresco and hence insists, as an image, on its iconicity. This shift from an object of science to an image as art is further marked by a shift in medium. The object's transformation into a photographic image points to how a specimen from medical history is itself staged, and to the genesis of this mise-en-scène in art. We encounter the production of an icon, one of the oldest forms of expression in painting. The icon exceeds painting itself: as the vera icon, which constitutes a testament, intending veracity and timelessness.

It is exactly this condition of signification which Anker exposes, in a medium which, as such, transmogrifies materials into its format, which vouches for authenticity: for example, the medium of photography. Anker's interventions in relation to a given image-context constitute a deviation from a given meaning, and at the same time, a deferral, delay in terms of forming new aspects of meaning immediately.[23] For this procedure, two further traits of her images are alienating ambiguity and atmospheric blurring.

These methods inhabit strategic functions; they disable the meaning that seems given, establishing a zone working against naïve claims for photographic authenticity. Both methods interfere with the image, replacing any authenticity in terms of the unambiguousness of the object with an uncertainty which may, at times, be unnerving. It is precisely in this undecidability where one encounters the potential to establish a site of reflection with regard to content – while the observer is challenged to evade habitual signification practices.

How, then, might the artistic habitus of these works be characterized? In terms of *The Glass Veil*, we might suggest that its intention can be comprehended if the images are approached in terms of the modalities of their appearance. That is, as mentioned, a shift in medium, gaze and the aspect of focus. For it is due to these elements that the observer no longer receives the information provided by the original objects. On the contrary, the images subject the observer to interrogation. Anker's methodology removes the prepared objects from the current leveling of historical narratives by silencing them, unlike the sciences. Such an immobilization[24] consequently removes the images from the means of the production of meaning and draws attention to the image as such. Suzanne Anker evokes a form of hesitation between image and meaning, producing a capability characteristic of stillness itself: to remove the image from narration in order to expose it – in and of itself.[25]

23 Stefan Germer has accurately pointed to the fact they might directly be characterized by means of Derrida's conception of différance. See Germer, "Rückblick nach vorn."

24 Regarding the relation between repetition and immobilization as elements constitutive to montage, see Giorgio Agamben, "Repetition and Stoppage: Guy Debord's Technique of Montage" In *Documenta X: Documents, vol. 2*, ed. Jean-François Chevrier (Ostfildern: Cantz, 1997), 72-75.

25 In terms of the removal of the narration, cf. ibid., 74.

IV. Synechein – The Art of Interweaving

"There is no seeing without thinking, but it is not sufficient to think in order to be able to see," Maurice Merleau-Ponty writes in *Eye and Mind.*[26] The philosopher subtly refers to questions which have for a long time pre-occupied researchers working in the neurosciences and cognitive sciences. Many questions are still unresolved: the questions of what perception is, of how, when and where it develops, of what the relation is between an 'internal sense of the image' and the perception of the outside world, of how brain activity is produced and what it signifies, beyond its measurability. In an interview with Susan Blackmore, the cognitive scientist Stuart Hameroff responds to the question of why sense perception is so difficult to describe as follows: "That's the hard problem. The brain is an excellent information processing system, but there's no accounting for how and why we have subjective experience, emotional feelings, an 'inner life'".[27] Hameroff addresses the problem in which the intricate relation of consciousness, body and perception is described as a fixed state for the purpose of clarifying what perception is. This means that there remain unresolved questions concerning the extent to which psychological and mental processes, or the relation between mental and physiological processes,[28] can be reduced to bio-chemical material causes. Can sensory perceptions be characterized as states and analyzed *eo ipso*? Presume that a sensory experience is not a given in relation to perception, but relies on intersubjective faculties and the qualia of a sensory experience. Hence subjective interiority is central to the installation *The Butterfly and the Brain* (2002) (See Dialogue II, fig. 28, pp. 88-89) and the video work *MRI Butterfly* (2008) (See Dialogue II, fig. 31, p. 95). The installation *The Butterfly and the Brain* consists of vitrines with objects such as optical devices, illustration charts of neurological diagrams and sculptural forms in wax which conflate brain coral with the morphology of the human brain. These images and objects engage with subjective identity and its apparent visualization by means of the imaging techniques used in the neurosciences.

Aside from the images which seem to be taken from the Rorschach test and objects in display cases, *Engram* (fig. 17) creates a significant relation to the neurosciences. The engram, from Greek for *en*, "into," and *gramma*, "inscription," refers to one of the traditional procedures of image production. It unites *ars* and

26 Maurice Merlau-Ponty, "Eye and Mind." In *The Primacy of Perception, and other essays on phenomenological psychology, the philosophy of art, history and politics*, ed. James Edie, (Evanston: Northwestern University Press, 1964).

27 Susan Blackmore, *Conversations on Concsciousness. What the best minds think about the brain, free will, and what it means to be human* (Oxford: Oxford University Press, 2006), 115.

28 If one has at least advanced to conceding that these are not states.

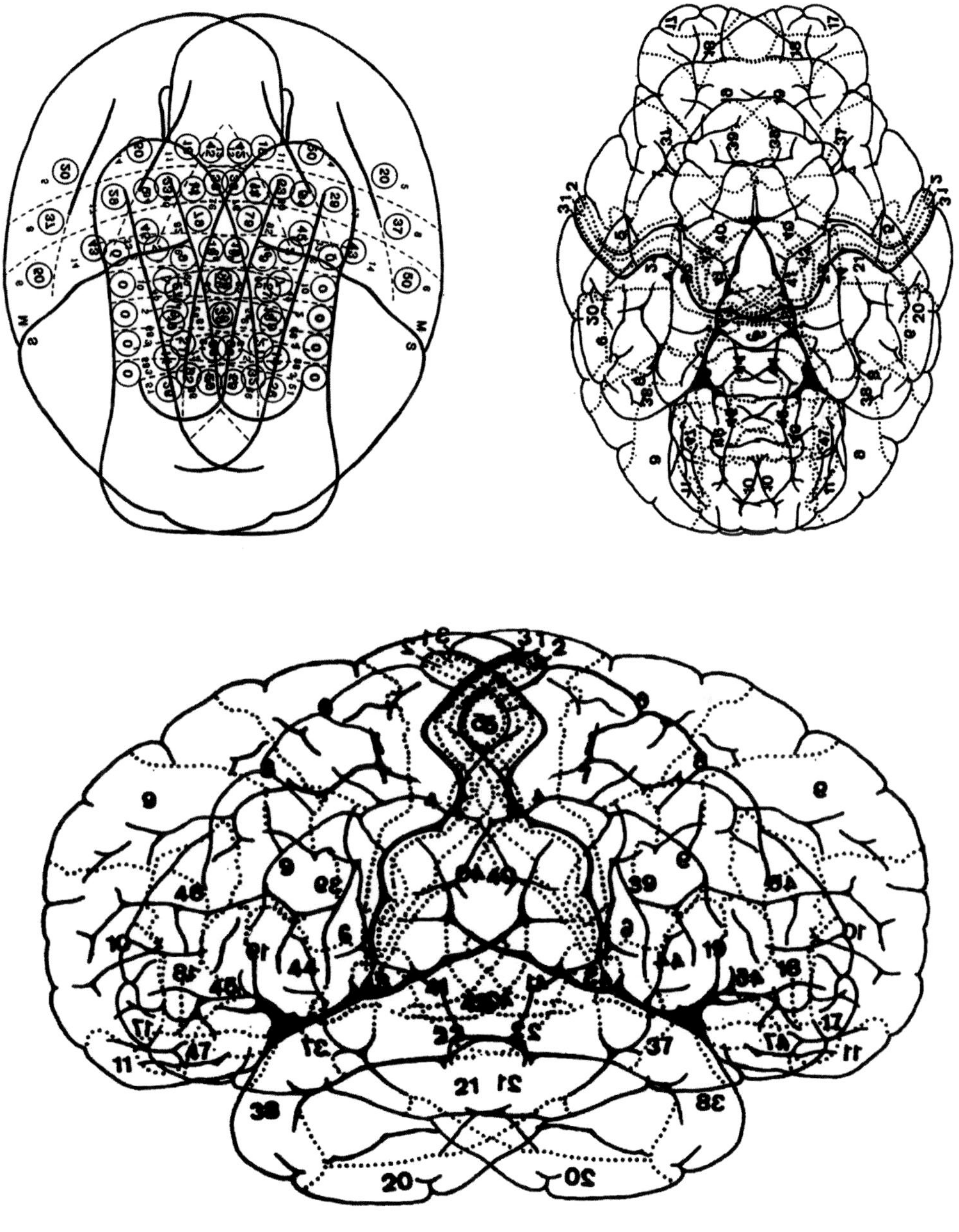

Figure 17. Theses images were derived from diagrams of the brain appropriated from neurology textbooks. Printed on transparent acetate and superimposed on one another, new representations such as Buddha, Scarab, and Yogi were created as part of *Engram* (2002).

techné–that is, art and craft. In the neurosciences, "engram" refers to a physiological trace or impression which leaves a stimulation effect, a memory, and which is a prevailing structural change within the brain. As an element of memory, an "engram" refers not only to what is past but also determines an individual's future actions. The concept intended through this designation, however, refers to art, more specifically to the link between ars and techné just mentioned. An engram is a kind of imprint. These images show the showing itself while reminding us of a determination of an image, which scientific images lack; it is evoked by means of the processuality of the indexicality deployed.[29]

The indexical impression of reality revealed in the image exposes it as an *ur-topos* of the image: as impression and trace. Its being is bound to reality in the form of testifying: that which it shows exists. A scientific image is certainly expected to refer to the original meaning of an image: as a state, the scientific image is to testify to its object being *exactly that*. But the principle of material context on which every imprint is based, in fact, testifies precisely not to similarity, for an *empreinte*[30] is more an "experiment of an uncertain outcome" than the erection of a "technical hypothesis in order to see what results from it."[31]

But the processuality of Anker's imprints renders possible an exposition of *difference*, an openness for possible metamorphoses. The creation of a replica no longer relies on similarity but becomes a paradigm of transformation. To produce an imprint implies fabricating a mesh of material relations from which the object emerges in the first place. These relations are also interwoven with abstract coordinates, myths, phantasms, knowledge and skill, etc. "Hence the imprint is simultaneously process and paradigm: it unites the two meanings of the word expérience–the scientific meaning of 'experiment' and the meaning of the 'recognition of the world'."[32]

Such an approach is further intensified in the video work *MRI Butterfly*. Since technologies such as MRI scans were first developed in the 1990s, there has been a persistent idea that not only can we observe brain activity in real time in the moving image, which is accurate, but we can also come to conclusions regarding a subject's individuality. In *MRI Butterfly*, fifteen apparently unspecific

29 The question whether a scientific image is to be understood as an imprint wherein the image shows that which is given or whether it is to be understood as a composition wherein the scientists leave their own traces is currently one of the most urgently discussed questions in the analysis of scientific images. For a recent contribution to the debate, see Lorraine Daston, "Bilder der Wahrheit, Bilder der Objektivität." In *Einbildungen: Interventionen*, ed, Jörg Huber (Zurich: Springer, 2005).

30 *Empreinte* is French term used in art theory meaning trace, mark, print or engram.

31 Georges Didi-Huberman, *Ähnlichkeit und Berührung: Archäologie, Anachronismus und Modernität des Abdrucks* (Cologne: DuMont, 1999), 17.

32 Even in the eighteenth century, experimental physics was an "experiential science".

yet identical brain scan images are juxtaposed with one another. On these scans we can also find the image of a small butterfly and an inkblot from a Rorschach test. The superimposition of Rorschach images, MRI scans and butterflies (See Dialogue II, figs. 32-33, pp. 96-97) create variations of figure-ground-constellations producing in the observer the optical illusion of the butterfly's movement and difference – while in fact the butterfly is identical in each image.

What does Suzanne Anker, then, show us through her work? As I suggest, she posits the question of what a manner of seeing is that continually oscillates between knowing and recognizing, between that which is given from the outside and that which appears from the inside. If the scientific image illuminates our perception, our thought processes and the relation between outer and inner images, then the artwork might be perceived as a form of research into perception at the same time as being recognized as art. In this sense, perception is both an epistemological method and an epistemological object. As the positing of a problem complex, perception is the process of the encounter of someone who perceives and something which appears. As a solution to a problem complex, as an epistemological path, however, it is the aesthetic experience of the artwork which appears.[33]

Furthermore, Anker connects the words 'known' and 'seeing' beyond the meaning of 'known' in the sense of 'being familiar'. 'Known' here explicitly demonstrates its etymological root, that of 'knowing' – as a form of *knowledge* – already connected to 'recognizing' – as a form of *perception*. Hence, testifying to the interweaving of knowledge and perception widens questions in terms of the theory of consciousness, concerning the "relation of 'inside' and 'outside', of one's 'own' and the 'alien', of 'seeing' and 'thinking.'"[34]

33 In this respect, I agree with Eva Schürmann: *Erscheinen und Wahrnehmen* (Munich: Wilhelm Fink, 2000), 15.

34 This equally addresses a circumstance relevant to the conception of the iconic episteme: what appears is the inner proximity between the imagination and the imago, the image. In this sense it is the imaginary as such which makes use of the interior sense of the image so as to create exteriorized images. The mental image and the *l'image objet* are two aspects of the same phenomenon; their difference, if there is any at all, consists in the fact that one of these images can be ephemeral, the other one durational, or, as described by Jacques Derrida and Bernard Stiegler in the *Échographies*: "L'image en général n'existe pas. Ce que l'on appelle l'image mentale et ce que j'appellerai ici l'image-objet, [...] sont deux faces d'un seul et même phénomène qui ne peuvent pas plus etre séparées [...]. La différence qui s'impose le plus immédiatement est que l'objective dure, tandis que la mentale est éphémère." Also see Thomas Macho, "Ist mir bekannt, dass ich sehe? Wittgensteins Frage nach dem inneren Sehen." In *Der zweite Blick. Bildgeschichte und Bildreflexion*, ed. Hans Belting et al. (Munich: Wilhelm Fink, 2000), 212.

Artistic research as perception in the aesthetic is consequently an interlocking of thought and vision.[35]

Hence it has for a significant period of time no longer been possible to consider the sciences and the arts as incommensurate fields. But this does not imply that the systems of knowledge marking them are identical and exchangeable. An approximation of the two disciplines ultimately require an attempt to contrast artistic and scientific methodologies. It is only then that we encounter intersection points of artistic and scientific conceptions. These nexus points generate the means by which epistemes of the arts can be uncovered. As I have suggested, this cannot be determined by means of resemblances, but rather through the recognition of non-convertible difference.

An artist's agency such as Suzanne Anker's researches the appearance, constitution and understanding of perception – concretely as art. Furthermore it produces perception, and this seems key: while we know that we perceive, we are not conscious of the modalities of our perception in the course of this act itself. Art shows us not only that we perceive but how we do so. It is exactly this doubling which is not determined through an actively participating subject – us. Rather, to think further, art determines our organization of perception if one recognizes an (art) image as a *Vor-bild* (in the German sense of pre-image and model) for attitudes and positionings in relation to visible reality.[36] It is exactly at this point where these images present eminent structural affinities between thought, sensory activity, the experience of perception and art observation itself. In the sense of the argument I have set forth, we can see how art is an ontological exception,[37] which does not symbolize but makes something present, presents something – *présente*: it is the appearance of perception. What is at stake is initially not to explain perception through other known faculties of consciousness, but to understand the perception of images as the form of perception unique and specific to art, the seeing-in[38]. Such a seeing-in raises the following question: what occurs within me when I see art? And seeing-in is, then, exactly the form of vision we encounter in relation to images. Human beings are not only capable of seeing something as something but have the extraordinary faculty of seeing something in something, and when this ability is employed, then, and only then, they see art.[39]

In his book *The Uses of Pleasure*, Michel Foucault poses an equally irritating and inspiring question, as to whether you can think, and thus perceive, differently

35 Cf. Schürmann, *Erscheinen und Wahrnehmen,* 93.

36 Lambert Wiesing, *Phänomene im Bild* (Munich: Wilhelm Fink, 2000), 20.

37 Ibid.

38 See: Rudolf Arnheim, *Visual Thinking* (Berkeley: University of California Press, 1969).

39 Also see Lambert Wiesing, *Das Mich der Wahrnehmung: Eine Autopsie* (Frankfurt am Main: Suhrkamp, 2009), 209.

from what you already think and perceive. Foucault answers this question with insistent affirmation and writes: "What use should the tenacity of knowledge have if it only brings with it the acquisition of knowledge, and does not to some extent and as far as possible prompt him who gains knowledge to err?" The reference to Foucault points to how there are repeating moments in life when the question of whether you can think differently from what you think, or perceive differently from what you see, is indispensable to looking or thinking further. In other words, Foucault is concerned with the critical work of thinking per se and hence – or so I would argue – with the extreme effort of knowing how and to what extent it is possible to think differently. As such he is intent on exploring what can be altered in your own thinking by venturing into an area of knowledge that is alien. Foucault defines this attempt as "the altered testing of one's own self and not as the simplifying appropriation of the other for the purposes of communication."[40] Exploring our knowledge systems enables us to experience the conditionality of knowledge in a different field. And, as such, you cannot respond to Foucault's question as to whether you can think differently from what you think, or perceive differently from what you perceive, with a simple "Yes!". Rather, you can enter into correspondence with him by responding to his interrogations with a reflection by Paul Valéry on the *specific* capacity of images and the arts. Sometimes, as Paul Valéry writes, an image articulates more than the thing it is portraying: "Une image est plus qu'une image et parfois plus que la chose même dont elle est image." What Paul Valéry describes is the additional value in every image, the additional value in art – which goes beyond the mere portrayal of the world. Fundamentally, for Valéry the focus is on the genuine and productive achievement of art itself, which in Suzanne Anker's work is described as a capacity which exceeds the mere depiction of the world. It is a matter then of opening up a dimension in which seeing itself is given an added visual value. Art does not necessarily depict the visible but, in addition, something not seen before. Artworks are investigations, laboratory experiments on the state and the responsibility of a subject for whom the work becomes a system of experiences and self-observations. Such is the work of Suzanne Anker.

40 Michel Foucault, *History of Sexuality. The Use of Pleasure,* vol. 2 (London: Vintage, 1990), 15-16.

References

Agamben, Giorgio. "Repetition and Stoppage: Guy Debord's Technique of Montage / Wiederholung und Stillstellung: zur Kompositionstechnik der Filme Guy Debords." In *Documenta X: Documents, vol. 2*, edited by Jean-François Chevrier, 68-75. Ostfildern: Cantz, 1997.

Anker, Suzanne, and Sabine Flach. "The Glass Veil." In *Habitas in Habitas: Emotion and Motion*, edited by Daniel Margulies, Jan Söffner and Sabine Flach, 141-158. Berlin : Peter Lang, 2010.

Arnheim, Rudolf. *Visual Thinking*. Berkeley: University of California Press, 1969.

Belting, Hans, and Dietmar Kamper. *Der zweite Blick: Bildgeschichte und Bildreflexion*, 211-229. München: Wilhelm Fink, 2000.

Benjamin, Walter. *Das Passagenwerk*, vol. 1, edited by Rolf Tiedemann, Frankfurt/Main: Suhrkamp, 1982.

Blackmore, Susan. *Conversations on Concsciousness. What the best minds think about the brain, free will, and what it means to be human*, Oxford: Oxford University Press, 2006.

Boehm, Gottfried. "Die Wiederkehr der Bilder." In *Was ist ein Bild?,* edited by Gottfried Boehm, Munich: Wilhelm Fink Verlag, 2006, 11-38.

Daston, Lorraine. "Bilder der Wahrheit, Bilder der Objektivität." In *Einbildungen: Interventionen*, edited by Jörg Huber, Zurich, Vienna: Springer, 2005, 117-154.

Didi-Huberman, Georges. *Ähnlichkeit und Berührung: Archäologie, Anachronismus und Modernität des Abdrucks*, Cologne: DuMont, 1999.

Flach, Sabine. *Körper-Szenarien: Zum Verhältnis von Körper und Bild in Videoinstallationen*, Munich: Wilhelm Fink, 2003.

Foucault, Michel. *History of Sexuality. The Use of Pleasure,* Vol. 2, London: Vintage, 1990.

Germer, Stefan. "Rückblick nach vorn." In *Jahresring 46. Germeriana Unveröffentlichte oder übersetzte Schriften von Stefan Germer zur zeitgenössischen und modernen Kunst*, edited by Julia Bernard, Cologne: DuMont, 1999, 86-103.

Heidegger, Martin. *Unterwegs zur Sprache*, Stuttgart: Klett-Cotta, 2007.

Kandinsky, Wassily. "Die Grundelemente der Form." In *Essays über Kunst und Künstler*, edited by Wassily Kandinsky, and Max Bill, Bern: Benteli, 1963, 71-73.

Khan-Magomedov, Selim. *Vhutemas: Moscou 1920-1930*, vol. 2, Paris: Editions du Regard, 1990.

Macho, Thomas. "Ist mir bekannt, dass ich sehe? Wittgensteins Frage nach dem inneren Sehen." In *Der zweite Blick. Bildgeschichte und Bildreflexion*, edited by Hans Belting, and Dietmar Kamper, Munich: Wilhelm Fink, 2000, 211-229.

Merlau-Ponty, Maurice. "Eye and Mind." In *The Primacy of Perception, and other essays on phenomenological psychology, the philosophy of art, history and politics*, edited by James Edie, Evanston: Northwestern University Press, 1964, 159-190.

Mitchell, William John Thomas. *Picture Theory: Essays on Verbal and Visual Representation*, Chicago: University of Chicago Press, 1994.

Plato. *Meno*, Stuttgart: Reclam, 2010.

Polanyi, Michael. *The Tacit Dimension*, Chicago: University of Chicago Press, 2009.

Schürmann, Eva. *Erscheinen und Wahrnehmen*, Munich: Wilhelm Fink, 2000.

Valéry, Paul. *Oeuvres*, vol. 1, Paris: Gallimard, 1990.

Warburg, Aby, Gertrud Bing, and Fritz Rougemont. *Gesammelte Schriften*. Leipzig: B.G. Teubner, 1932.

Warnke, Martin. *Politische Landschaft. Zur Kunstgeschichte der Natur*, Munich, Vienna: Hanser, 1992.

Weigel, Sigrid. "Bilder als Hauptakteure auf dem Schauplatz der Erkenntnis. Zur poiesis und episteme sprachlicher und visueller Bilder." In *Ästhetik – Erfahrung : Interventionen*, edited by Wlad Godzich and Jörg Huber, 191-212. Zürich: Springer, 2004.

Wiesing, Lambert. *Phänomene im Bild*, Munich: Wilhelm Fink, 2000.

Wiesing, Lambert. "Vom Ich zum Mich der Wahrnehmung: eine Verstrickung." In *Ich – der Einzelne in seinen Netzen*, edited by Konrad Paul Liessmann, Vienna: Zsolnay, 2014, 204-230.

Wittgenstein, Ludwig. *Vermischte Bemerkungen. Eine Auswahl aus dem Nachlass*, edited by Georg Henrik von Wright, Frankfurt/Main: Suhrkamp, 1994.

List of Illustrations

Fig. 17: Top left: Suzanne Anker, *Engram* series *#4*, 2002. Archival inkjet print on paper, 8.5 x 11 in (21.6 x 28 cm); Top right: Suzanne Anker, *Engram* series *#9*, 2002. Archival inkjet print on paper, 8.5 x 11 in (21.6 x 28 cm); Bottom: Suzanne Anker, *Engram* series *#5*, 2002. Archival inkjet print on paper, 8.5 x 11 in (21.6 x 28 cm).

2. Dialogues

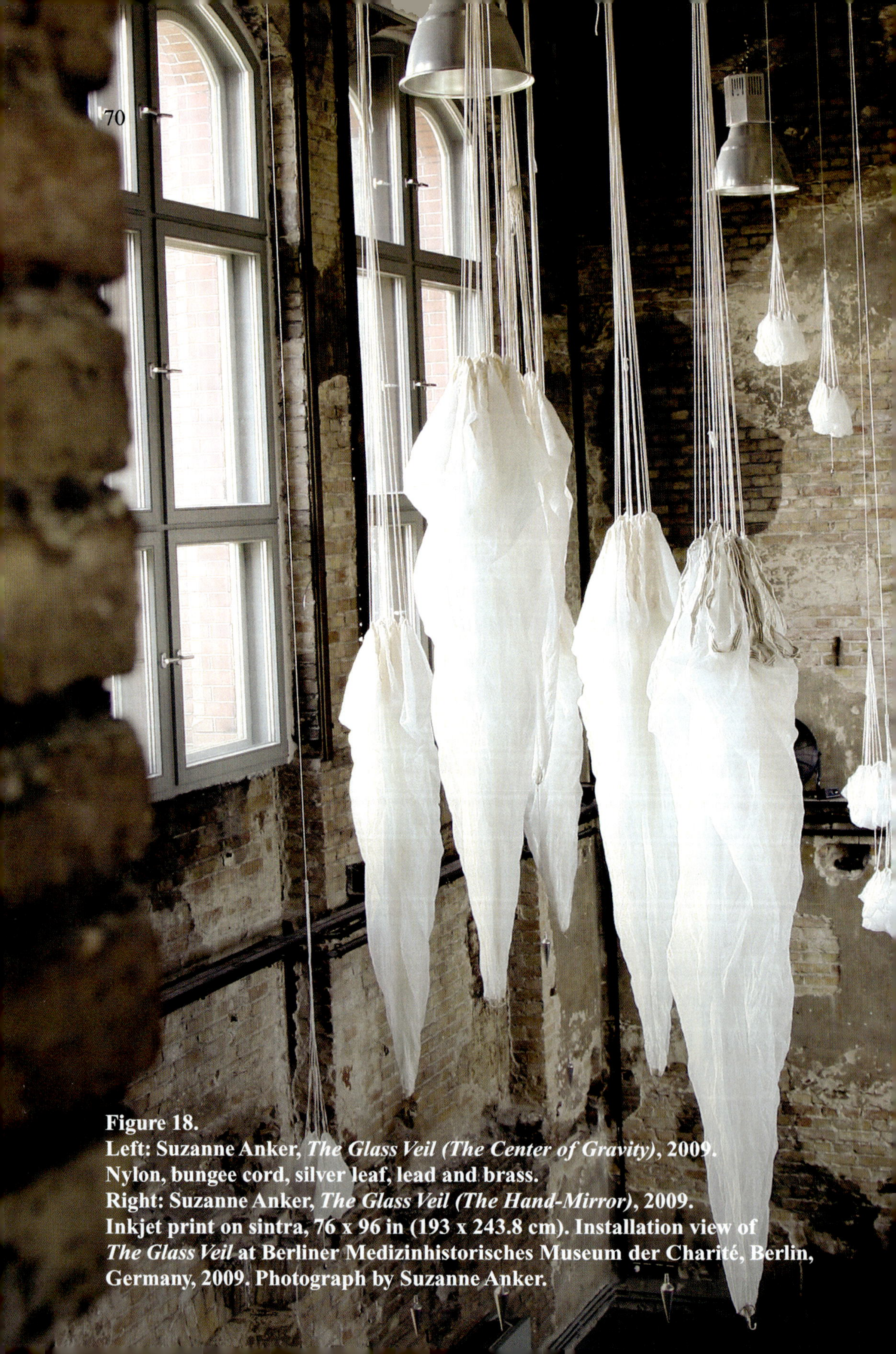

Figure 18.
Left: Suzanne Anker, *The Glass Veil (The Center of Gravity)*, 2009. Nylon, bungee cord, silver leaf, lead and brass.
Right: Suzanne Anker, *The Glass Veil (The Hand-Mirror)*, 2009. Inkjet print on sintra, 76 x 96 in (193 x 243.8 cm). Installation view of *The Glass Veil* at Berliner Medizinhistorisches Museum der Charité, Berlin, Germany, 2009. Photograph by Suzanne Anker.

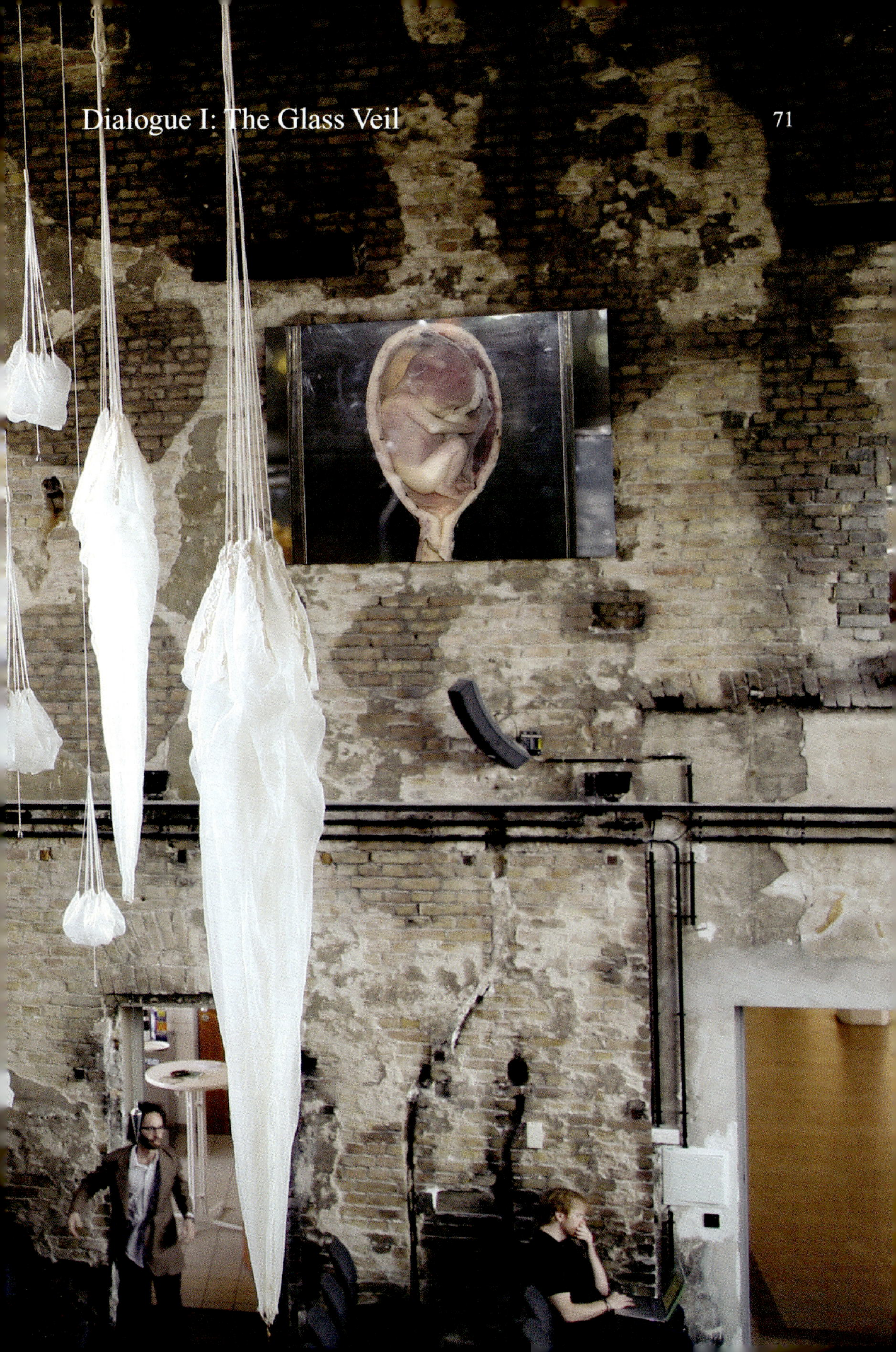

Dialogue I: The Glass Veil

Suzanne Anker & Sabine Flach

Sabine Flach: In *The Glass Veil* project (fig. 18) as well as other work, you employ objects, materials and topics that are already given. In other words, the subjects of your work previously exist, in other spaces and for alternate reasons. In essence, you are not the absolute provenance of your images. Could you describe how you see your work with regard to such matters?

Suzanne Anker: Suspended in liquid-filled vessels and aligned as a display, human specimens in medical museums are, readymade sources of wonder. Within the genre of *nature morte*, these photographs spotlight various visual perspectives and illuminating reflections. I look for germane details, particulars which had not been accounted for by the museum curators or staff. For example, in *The Hand-Mirror* (fig. 19), traces of human fingerprints mark the cases' transparent surface. There are also "swish" marks left behind by the janitor's hand movements during the process of cleaning the façade. These on-site artifacts alter the meanings of the long-established arrays of specimens. When such residua are incorporated into a photographic image they become a form of added value. My work with these extant collections is a translation of preserved specimens into emotive and striking images. However some of the representations such as "babies in bottles" remain highly charged personifications. Imagine a person trying to get closer to a specimen, endeavoring to reach out and touch it, only to find that it is not within reach. Like death itself, there is a barrier obscuring what is possible to grasp.

SF: With reference to the previous question, please talk about how, why and in which ways you make aesthetic decisions. What specific characteristics of these objects allow you to convert them into works of art?

SA: When I set out to conduct a photographic project, I visit the prospective site and peruse what is there. I then return to specific objects which for formal or idiosyncratic reasons I find compelling. Is color being phenomenologically expressed? Is light reflected or refracted to produce multiplied views? Are there details of the specimen that can stand alone as an image? This is a process that permits me to put my *imprimatur* on the already given. It becomes a signatory process that transforms such objects from clinical artifacts into somatic phenomena. Meaning and content are transposed, not so much by context but by superimposition of a subjective self, a way of seeing.

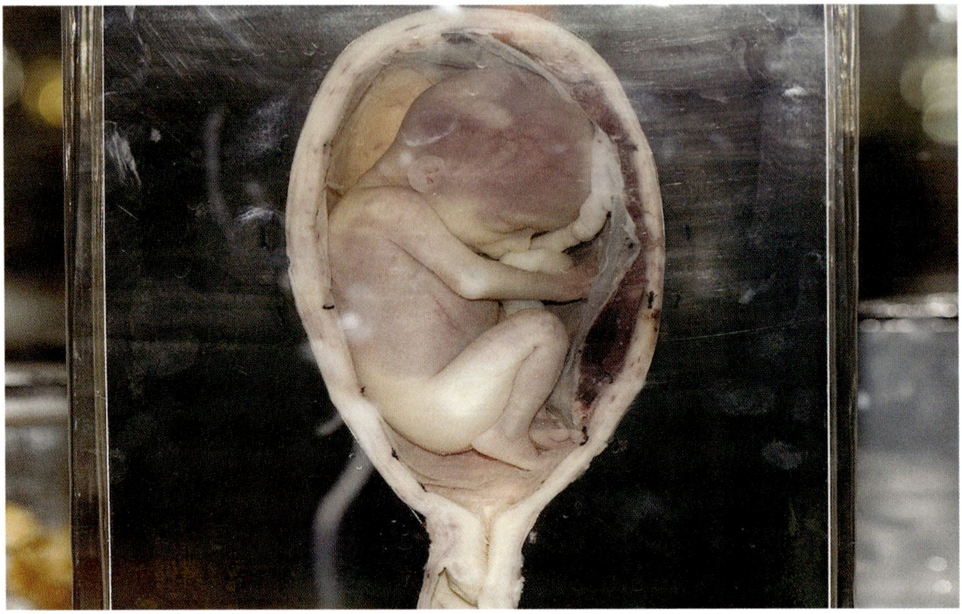

Figure 19. Suzanne Anker, *The Glass Veil (The Hand-Mirror)*, 2009.
Inkjet print on sintra, 76 x 96 in (193 x 243.8 cm).

SF: A number of contemporary artists incorporate concepts associated with the natural world in their work. For example, Mark Dion's *Systema Metropolis* exhibition at London's Natural History Museum in 2007 or his piece for dOCUMENTA (13) in Kassel, which we both saw. The late Helen Chadwick is another example. Other artists work with existing collections, or with the historical concept of *Wunderkammer*. You are especially interested in medical history museums. Could we please talk a bit about this development and your interest in specimens and medical objects?

SA: Both Mark Dion's and the late Helen Chadwick's work are both significant examples of the intersections between the natural and cultural worlds. Dion mixes natural history with consumer culture while Chadwick's work is concerned with human and animal bodies as subject matter. Both artists cross the diminishing barriers of the nature/culture divide in their work.

I echo the same diffusion in my work as the natural world is subsumed and integrated into the cultural coordinates of display. My interest in medical museums arose out of my travels to Europe and a photographic turn in my work. I had not been exposed to medical specimens or such museums in the United States, although there are some, most notably the Mütter Museum. The Mütter Museum had been already incorporated into art practice by several artists, so I considered it off limits as an institutional site. After viewing these historical collections in Europe, countless questions filled my thoughts. Viewing human body parts or fetuses immersed in glass containers is, of course, an intense experience. These vessels are in some ways like transparent graveyards dressed as historical relics. They are suspended in time. Are they artifacts, objects or merely human remains? They pose acute problems for language. They signify ambiguity–"an uncertainty or inexactness of meaning in language"–as the dictionary recounts as its definition. Such indeterminateness surrounds these objects, which is both unnerving and at the same time poses revealing questions about our relationship towards expression and emotion.

SF: With respect to *The Glass Veil* exhibition, which took place in the enormous Lecture Hall Ruin at the Charité Medical Museum in Berlin in 2009, how would you describe your process of "sense-making"?

SA: My process of "sense-making" reflects Roman Jakobson's theories of how communication functions but with one caveat: the intervention of polysemous and multi-coded clues. As a noteworthy linguist, his theory of communication is elegant and straightforward. He describes the process of communication as a six part system in which he differentiates the elements: 1) context; 2) speaker; 3) receiver; 4) contact between the two; 5) common code; 6) message[1]. What occurs in multi-coded or indeterminate systems is not as succinct. Since aesthetic interpretation relies so heavily on disparate pairing and multi-layered metaphors, single interpretations are rarely fully achieved, never fully exposed. This form of semiosis is rife with error and contradiction, which in art practice is the point. Art is a realm of communication that embodies various underlying suppositions concerning the receiver, which play a significant interpretive role. Already inherent within the receiver's data bank of understanding are in-bred propositions, value-laden assumptions, and experiential reverberations. This idea has been broadly noted within discussions of modern and, particularly, contemporary art.

For a general public, images of fetuses are intensely recognizable icons producing immediate and provocative responses. From shock to pathos, from disquietude to sheer awe, the fetus is a universal marvel. Sometimes viewers ponder the why, when and how this human specimen came to be on display, and, at other times, they express dismay or downright anger. As devices of inquiry, these images pierce the viewer's memory reservoirs, setting off a cascade of thoughts and feelings based on psychological factors, religious values, and educational backgrounds. Family beliefs, issues of privacy and public decency are also some of the concerns evoked.

1 Roman Jakobson, Krystyna Pomorska, and Stephen Rudy. *Verbal Art, Verbal Sign, Verbal Time* (Minneapolis: University of Minnesota Press, 1985).

Other aspects of "sense-making" in my work rely on self-expression and self-reflection, both of which are necessary components for a work to transmit emotion. Recurrent images in an artist's body of work are quite common over the course of a career. Such reworking is not necessarily because the artist does not engage new subject matter, but because these images are seldom fully exhausted. Each trial attempts to draw out another dimension of what has already been articulated. The image of the fetus has been part of my work since 1969, after I gave birth to my daughter.

SF: Your installation in the Lecture Hall Ruin incorporated upside down parachutes as spatial markers, integral with a sense of movement. What is the significance of the parachutes in such a setting?

SA: As you are well aware of, the Lecture Hall Ruin is not a neutral space. Left in the form of a bombed out site, it speaks to the memory of World War II. It is a place that was formerly a lecture hall in which medical issues concerning pathology were discussed and debated. At that time, it was named the Rudolf Virchow Lecture Hall, after the physician known as the father of pathology. Virchow (1821-1902) was also an anthropologist and politician dedicated to public health. It is worth noting that such an eminent researcher and scholar, ironically, did not believe in Darwin's theory of evolution, not because of religious faith, but because he considered it highly improbable.[2]

SF: Collections are "sites of knowledge production" where "epistemic objects" – as the historian of science Hans-Jörg Rheinberger refers to them – open a nexus to fields of inquiry. Is specific knowledge produced by investigating collections? Where do you see your work in this regard?

SA: Collections of objects carry with them silent conversations. They speak without brains or mouths but by cerebrally or sensually interacting with the viewer's perception and memories. Aesthetic decisions as well, are in many cases similarly unconscious and not conceivable through language. When I met Hans-Jörg Rheinberger, he maintained that he did not consider art to be an "epistemic object." He justified his analysis in terms of data sets related to scientific research. Although some cultural historians have endorsed this term as it relates to art, he has not advocated such cultural applications of his theories. This is also true of others – Jean Baudrillard and his concept of *simulacra* in the 1980s is another case

2 Abraham Jacobi, *Rudolf Virchow: An address introductory to the course of lectures of the term 1881-1882* (Paris: BIUM, 2010).

in point. When Baudrillard attended one of my Thanksgiving dinners in New York City, he was bemused by the fact that his theories had migrated into art, particularly neo-geo and appropriation art. He staunchly commented that none of these art practices pertained to his post-structuralist theories. I remain convinced that art objects are epistemic, encompassing all of the surrounding processes, materials and concepts related to their constitution and consumption. If one proceeds to deconstruct the encircling structures that privilege art objects' fabrication, one is confronted with material, social, economic and political considerations in addition to its aesthetic parameters. Art objects are both material markers of memory and physical remainders of time periods, which in turn assimilate ideas and constraints of particular epochs.

SF: You have had access to several historical medical museums. Medical museums are places that store archives and specimens for research purposes. How would you therefore relate your work to current developments of "artistic knowledge production"?

SA: "Artistic knowledge production" is a term rarely used to describe art practice in America. The art object in America is to a disturbing degree driven by consumer culture, as a vehicle towards celebrity status – for the artist, collector and institution. My work generally moves outside the traditional boundaries of market-driven economies, and instead, transgresses, trespasses and intersects with several distinct disciplines: art history and theory, the history of biology and its laboratory practices as well as cultural criticism. Art as a knowledge-producing process can be apprehended as a reflection of the values in a society, or as a provisional method of innovation. However, that requires uncensored criticism, historical knowledge and a skeptical awareness of institutional support structures. If one believes that "curatorial nannies" or "tax-deduction incentives" are the prime arbiters of culture, then the *art game* is set as is. For art to be a knowledge-producing process it is compelled to operate within an experimental system where outcomes are initially unknown. It must bring to the fore otherwise unexpected interconnections that reinforce desired values supporting a knowledge-based society.

Historical medical museums, or museums in general, create conditions of display which put forward a proposition. All exhibitions are programs with coded messages and discrete points of view. It is within this realm that a curator has an opportunity to forge a dialogue with the public, protect and catalogue "material culture" and formulate some kind of historical trajectory concerning practices and methods. This is true for medical museums as well as art museums, although in medical museums preserved fragments of human bodies, or as in this case preserved fetuses as specimens, are on display.

SF: As an artist, what kind of "knowledge" do you explore in terms of the specific ways of working with these specimens?

SA: The preserved specimens remain artifacts of social, economic, political and medical power. Originally employed as teaching aides for the medical sciences or collected as rarefied if not eccentric quarry in *Wunderkammer,* the specimen is a form of time capsule. Institutions seriously regard their importance as documentary evidence of historical and medical value.[3] These highly charged specimens pose numerous and diverse questions: Where did they come from? What economic and social classes do they represent? Why are they discomforting to gaze at, yet at the same time possess a sublime beauty? What were the preservation techniques used? Are these methods still in use? Who posed the "babies in bottles"? Were these fetuses taken from unwed mothers? Why don't we see these kinds of specimens more regularly in America? The cultural and social issues surrounding these entities make them epistemic objects – objects that generate knowledge. In addition, recent discourse into the medical humanities suggests a link between these "samples" and the emergent field of biobanking.[4] For example, umbilical cords which were once considered abject and disposable are now biobanked for future use. Precious stem cells can be extracted from this "organ" with the hope that one day they will be useful as a repair kit for offspring or for a related family member in need of donor matches.

SF: You titled your series of work from the Museum Vrolik Academic Medical Center *Water Babies* (2004) (figs. 20-21). What relation does this series have to the 19th century novel by Charles Kingsley, which bears the same name?

SA: Charles Kingsley, a 19th century Anglican theologian and friend of Charles Darwin, believed that "moral lessons of nature" could be taught through his delightful fairy tale *The Water-Babies*[5] (fig. 22). In this parable, which was read out loud to children in Victorian England, a young chimney sweep, Tom, appears filthy and uncouth, a clear indication of his lowly status. In an effort to escape his master and others running after him, he jumps into a stream where he falls into a deep sleep. Here he meets up with the fairies that turn him into a water baby.

3 Samuel Alberti and Elizabeth Hallam, *Medical Museums: Past, Present, Future* (London: Royal College of Surgeons of England, 2013).

4 Karin Tybjerg, "From Bottled Babies to Biobanks: Anatomical Collections in the 21st Century." In *The Fate of Anatomical Collections*, ed. Rina Knoeff et al. (Farnham: Ashgate, 2015).

5 This popular story was read to children in England as a moral warning. For others, it was interpreted as a reconciliation of Darwin's theory of evolution with theological perspectives on embryology.

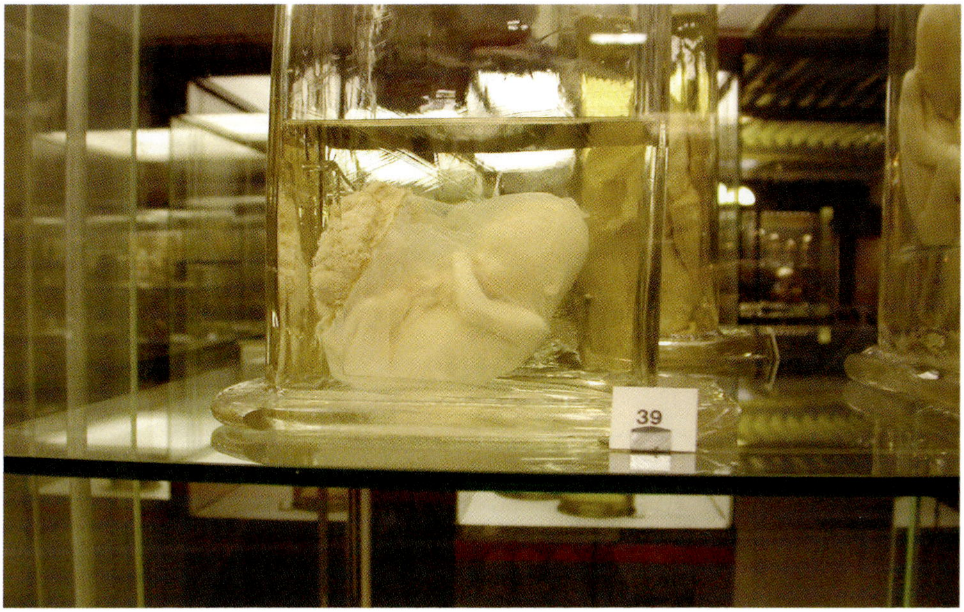

Figure 20. Suzanne Anker, *Water Babies (Veil)*, 2004.
Archival inkjet print on paper, 24 x 36 in (60.9 x 91.4 cm).

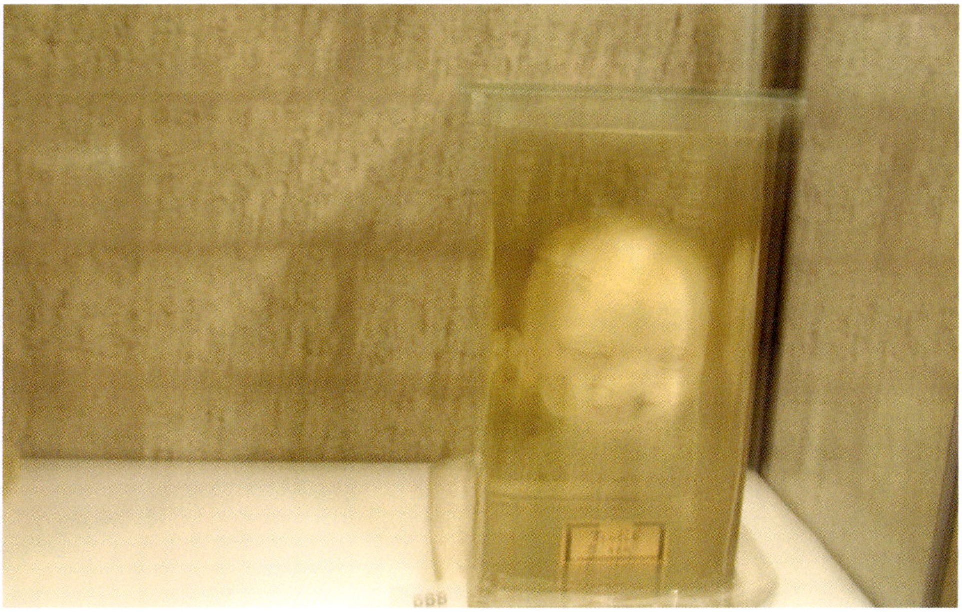

Figure 21. Suzanne Anker, *Water Babies (Mask)*, 2004.
Archival inkjet print on paper, 24 x 36 in (60.9 x 91.4 cm).

In this physical state he develops a set of gills. As he learns through reason and judgment to accomplish the tasks before him, he changes once again. Each time he performs his cerebral missions he ascends the phylogenetic order from fish to amphibian to mammal.

In an effort to reconcile Darwin's theory of evolution with Christian theology, Kingsley sets up a dialogue between Tom and one of the Chief Fairies Mother Carey. Encountering her, Tom queries:

> I hear you are very busy.
> I am never more busy than I am now, she said without stirring a finger.
> I heard ma'am, that you were always making new beasts out of old.
> So people fancy. But I am not going to trouble myself to make things, my little dear.
> I sit here and make them make themselves.

Ironically, Mother Carey's words resonate not only with Darwin's tangled bank of endless forms, but also preface current scientific experiments, particularly with glowing green monkeys. As Maggie Fox of Reuters reported in 2009: "Japanese researchers have genetically engineered monkeys whose hair roots, skin and blood glow green under a special light, and who have passed on their traits to their offspring, the first time this has been achieved in a primate."[6] What is important in this experiment is that "green glowing monkeys have green-glowing babies." So, as Mother Carey states: "I sit here and make them make themselves."

In this photographic set taking its title from Kingsley's parable, the viewer is confronted with fetuses submerged in liquid. Akin to an aquarium, these images are not of the imagination. In zones of ambiguity, bodies and their parts float anonymously as mementos marking historical time. In an ocular joust, the observer assumes a pose, as details of his gaze achieve focus. Thoughts of definition enter and exit the viewer's consciousness until some determination of meaning, however tentative, appears. At the same time the glass becomes a mirror of our concealed selves, as we spy on inscrutable worlds of the unborn and the undead. Occupying a world of unimaginable repose, a fetus is a primal marvel. A mystery in itself, the fetus has come to represent life as a continuous cycle moving from birth to death, an unfolding of a single cell that has within its code an expiration date.

SF: You have investigated the collections residing in three medical museums: the Charité - Universitätsmedizin in Berlin, the Museum Vrolik Academic Medical Center in Amsterdam, and the Medical Museion in Copenhagen. How do you compare your experiences with each venue?

---

6 Maggie Fox, "Green-glowing monkeys have green glowing babies." *Reuters*, May 27, 2009.

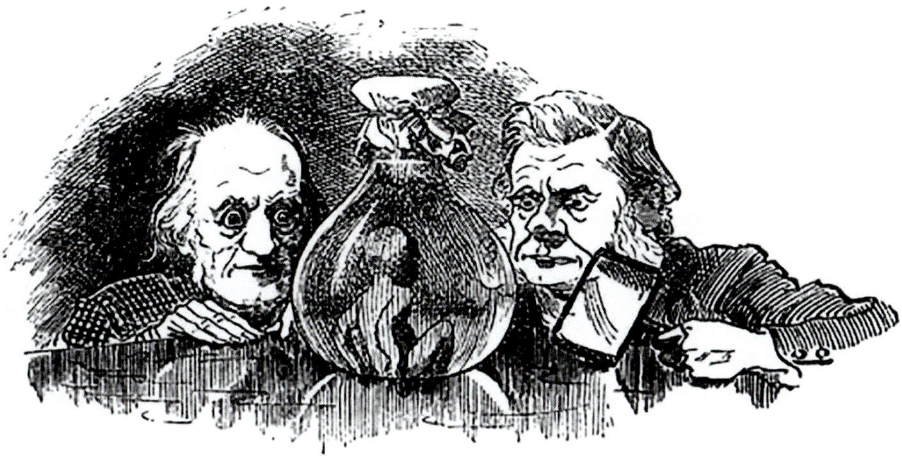

Figure 22. Richard Owen (left) and Thomas Henry Huxley inspect a "water baby" in Edward Linley Sambourne's 1885 illustration.

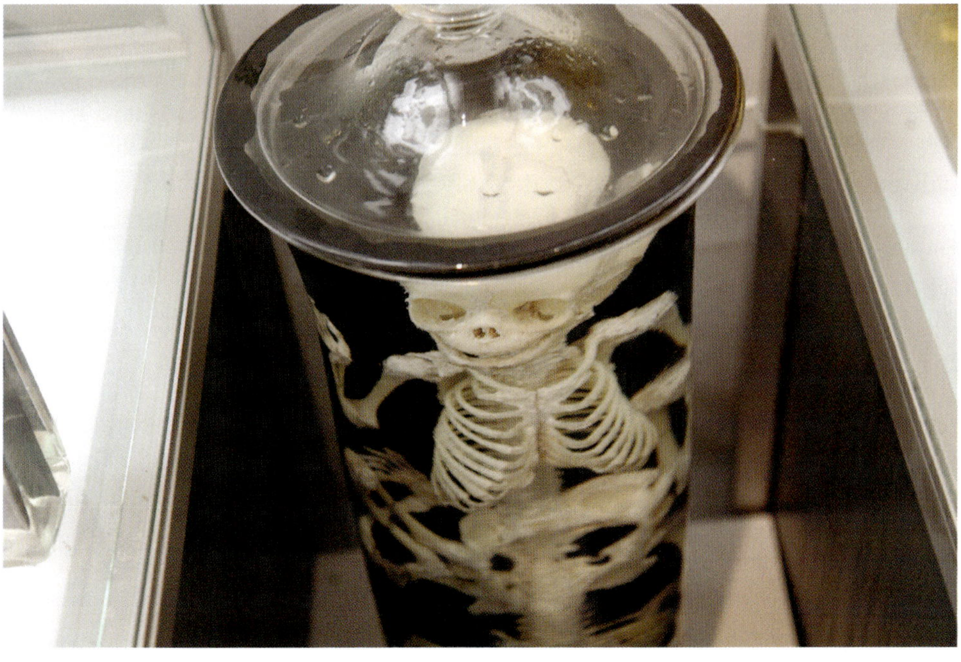

Figure 23. Suzanne Anker, *Sons and Daughters (Skeleton Jar)*, 2010.
Archival inkjet print on paper, 24 x 36 in (60.9 x 91.4 cm).

SA: Of course there are many differences and similarities as in all collections and museums, and I cannot comment in any scholarly way in assessing these holdings. Each institution has a unique history dependent in part on specific cultural considerations and missions. In each space, various forms of access was available or sanctioned. By comparing the three photographic sets, *The Glass Veil* (figs. 18, 19), *Water Babies* (figs. 20, 21), and *Sons and Daughters* (figs. 23-27) it is evident that each set embeds a distinct consciousness. In *Water Babies*, there is a feeling of the fleeting moment, captured by an out of focus camera lens and an array of monochromatic hues of ochre: the stucco walls, fluorescent lights and specimen skins. In *The Glass Veil*, scale becomes the arbiter of experience, as the viewer is dwarfed by the historic Lecture Hall Ruin's space. In *Sons and Daughters*, human remains present themselves as fetish-like objects invoking an anthropological gaze. In each case, the "remains" themselves trump any articulation of clarity. Where the specimens, or shall I say artifacts, are concerned, analytic processes and procedures such as measurement, age or location can be calculated, recorded and archived. Such is the nature of modes of investigation. But such rational systems of analysis do not apply to emotions and their somatic fallout.

SF: Interpreting visualizing processes is a parameter of "subjective seeing." What relevance do visualization techniques have for you?

SA: Visualizing these specimens through a barrier, a glass, a camera, and a lens creates a distancing frame of reference. These barriers bring into play the environmental conditions affecting objects in distinct spaces. Because I have neither touched the specimens in the jars, nor opened them nor repositioned them, I can only apprehend them indirectly. Redressing them in this way, I only know them speculatively, not empirically or first-hand. They are protected from me and I from them, from fear, from disgust, from anguish.

SF: Do the modes or processes of transgression and transformation play a role in your work and if so, how?

SA: I would say that a portion of my work is transgressive in that it exposes concepts regarding human vulnerability: disease, malformation, and death. These are concepts that are accessed in many forms of art: theater, music, literature, film. However, certain understandings and their related images are more jarring when presented large-scale and up close. In their stillness they speak to a disquieting quietude while in suffused repose. That is their power. In many ways they are trophies of life's transience. As noted by poet Anne Sexton:

Somebody who should have been born
is gone.

Just as the earth puckered its mouth,
each bud puffing out from its knot,
I changed my shoes, and then drove south.

Up past the Blue Mountains, where
Pennsylvania humps on endlessly,
wearing, like a crayoned cat, its green hair,

its roads sunken in like a gray washboard;
where, in truth, the ground cracks evilly,
a dark socket from which the coal has poured,

Somebody who should have been born
is gone.

the grass as bristly and stout as chives,
and me wondering when the ground would break,
and me wondering how anything fragile survives;

up in Pennsylvania, I met a little man,
not Rumpelstiltskin, at all, at all…
he took the fullness that love began.

Returning north, even the sky grew thin
like a high window looking nowhere.
The road was as flat as a sheet of tin.

Somebody who should have been born
is gone.

Yes, woman, such logic will lead
to loss without death. Or say what you meant,
you coward… this baby that I bleed.

"The Abortion" from *All My Pretty Ones* by Anne Sexton. Copyright © 1962 by Anne Sexton, renewed 1990 by Linda G. Sexton. Reprinted by permission of Houghton Mifflin Harcourt Publishing Company. All rights reserved.

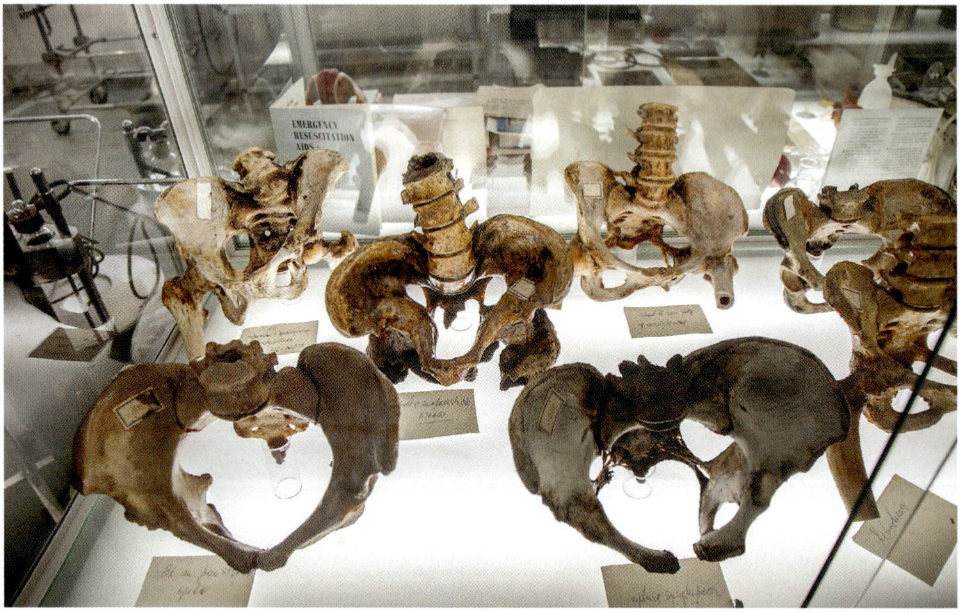

Figure 24. Suzanne Anker, *Sons and Daughters (Pelvis)*, 2010.
Archival inkjet print on paper, 24 x 36 in (60.9 x 91.4 cm).

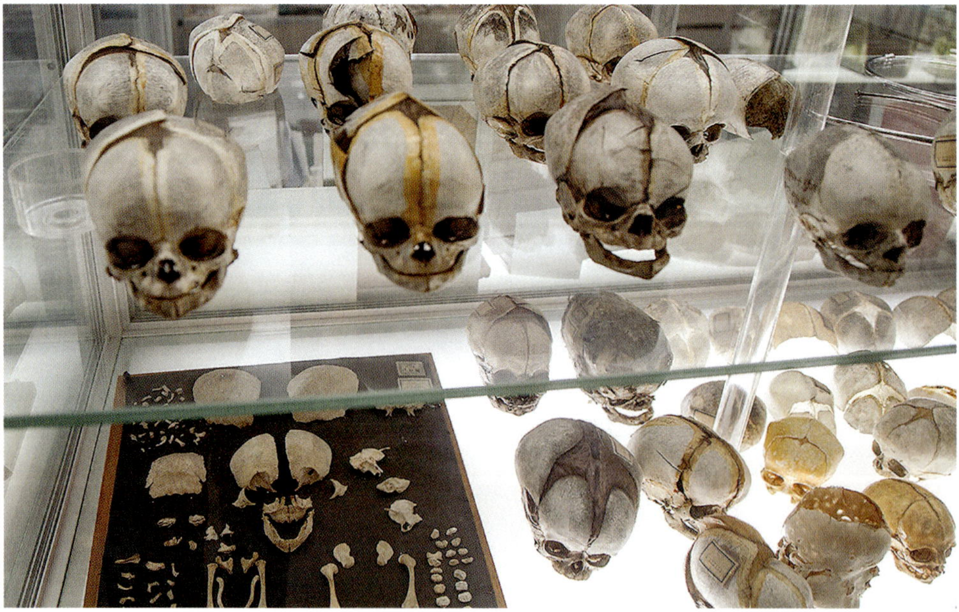

Figure 25. Suzanne Anker, *Sons and Daughters (Fetish)*, 2010.
Archival inkjet print on paper, 24 x 36 in (60.9 x 91.4 cm).

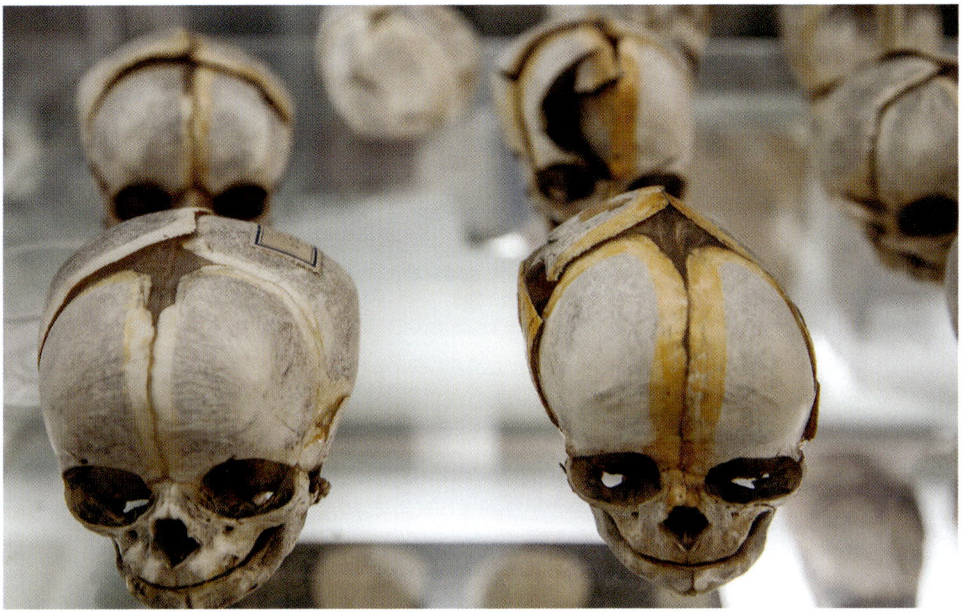

Figure 26. Suzanne Anker, *Sons and Daughters (Cranial Winds)*, 2010.
Archival inkjet print on paper, 24 x 36 in (60.9 x 91.4 cm).

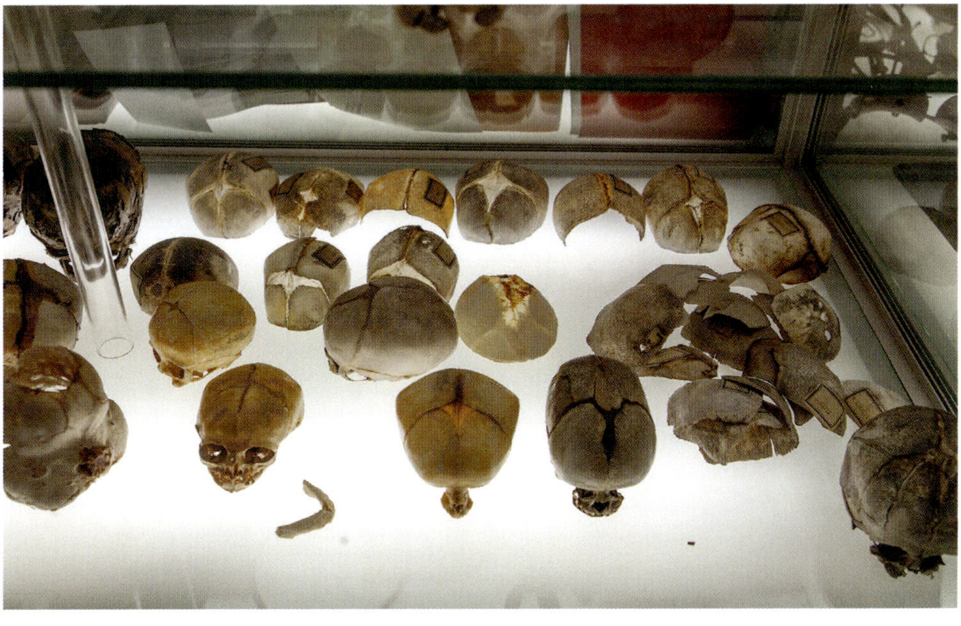

Figure 27. Suzanne Anker, *Sons and Daughters (Evolution)*, 2010.
Archival inkjet print on paper, 24 x 36 in (60.9 x 91.4 cm).

References

Alberti, Samuel J. M. M., and Elizabeth Hallam. *Medical Museums: Past, Present, Future*. London: Royal College of Surgeons of England, 2013.
Baudrillard, Jean. *Simulacra and simulation*. Ann Arbor: University of Michigan Press, 1994.
Fox, Maggie. "Green-glowing monkeys have green glowing babies." *Reuters*, May 27, 2009. http://www.reuters.com/article/2009/05/27/us-monkeys-green-idUSTRE54Q4A520090527.
Jacobi, Abraham. *Rudolf Virchow: An address introductory to the course of lectures of the term 1881-1882*. Paris: BIUM, 2010.
Jakobson, Roman, Krystyna Pomorska, and Stephen Rudy. *Verbal Art, Verbal Sign, Verbal Time*. Minneapolis: University of Minnesota Press, 1985.
Kingsley, Charles. *The Water-Babies: A Fairy-Tale for a Land-Baby*. London: Puffin, 1994.
Rheinberger, Hans-Jorg. *An Epistemology of the Concrete: Twentieth- Century Histories of Life*. Duke University Press Books, 2010.
Sexton, Anne. *All My Pretty Ones*. Boston: Houghton Mifflin Harcourt, 1962.
Tybjerg, Karin. "From Bottled Babies to Biobanks: Anatomical Collections in the 21st Century." In *The Fate of Anatomical Collections*, edited by Rina Knoeff and Robert Zwijnenberg. Farnham, Surrey: Ashgate, 2015.

List of Illustrations

Fig. 18: Left: Suzanne Anker, *The Glass Veil (The Center of Gravity),* 2009. Nylon, bungee cord, silver leaf, lead and brass. Right: Suzanne Anker, *The Glass Veil (The Hand-Mirror),* 2009. Inkjet print on sintra, 76 x 96 in (193 x 243.8 cm). Installation view of *The Glass Veil* at Berliner Medizinhistorisches Museum der Charité, Berlin, Germany, 2009. Photograph by Suzanne Anker.
Fig. 19: Suzanne Anker, *The Glass Veil (The Hand-Mirror)*, 2009. Inkjet print on sintra, 76 x 96 in (193 x 243.8 cm).
Fig. 20: Suzanne Anker, *Water Babies (Veil)*, 2004. Archival inkjet print on paper, 24 x 36 in (60.9 x 91.4 cm).
Fig. 21: Suzanne Anker, *Water Babies (Mask)*, 2004. Archival inkjet print on paper, 24 x 36 in (60.9 x 91.4 cm).
Fig. 22: Linley Sambourne, *Richard Owen and Thomas Henry Huxley inspect a water baby*, 1885. Illustration.
Fig. 23: Suzanne Anker, *Sons and Daughters (Skeleton Jar)*, 2010. Archival inkjet print on paper, 24 x 36 in (60.9 x 91.4 cm).
Fig. 24: Suzanne Anker, *Sons and Daughters (Pelvis)*, 2010. Archival inkjet print on paper, 24 x 36 in (60.9 x 91.4 cm).
Fig. 25: Suzanne Anker, *Sons and Daughters (Fetish)*, 2010. Archival inkjet print on paper, 24 x 36 in (60.9 x 91.4 cm).
Fig. 26: Suzanne Anker, *Sons and Daughters (Cranial Winds)*, 2010. Archival inkjet print on paper, 24 x 36 in (60.9 x 91.4 cm).
Fig. 27: Suzanne Anker, *Sons and Daughters (Evolution)*, 2010. Archival inkjet print on paper, 24 x 36 in (60.9 x 91.4 cm).

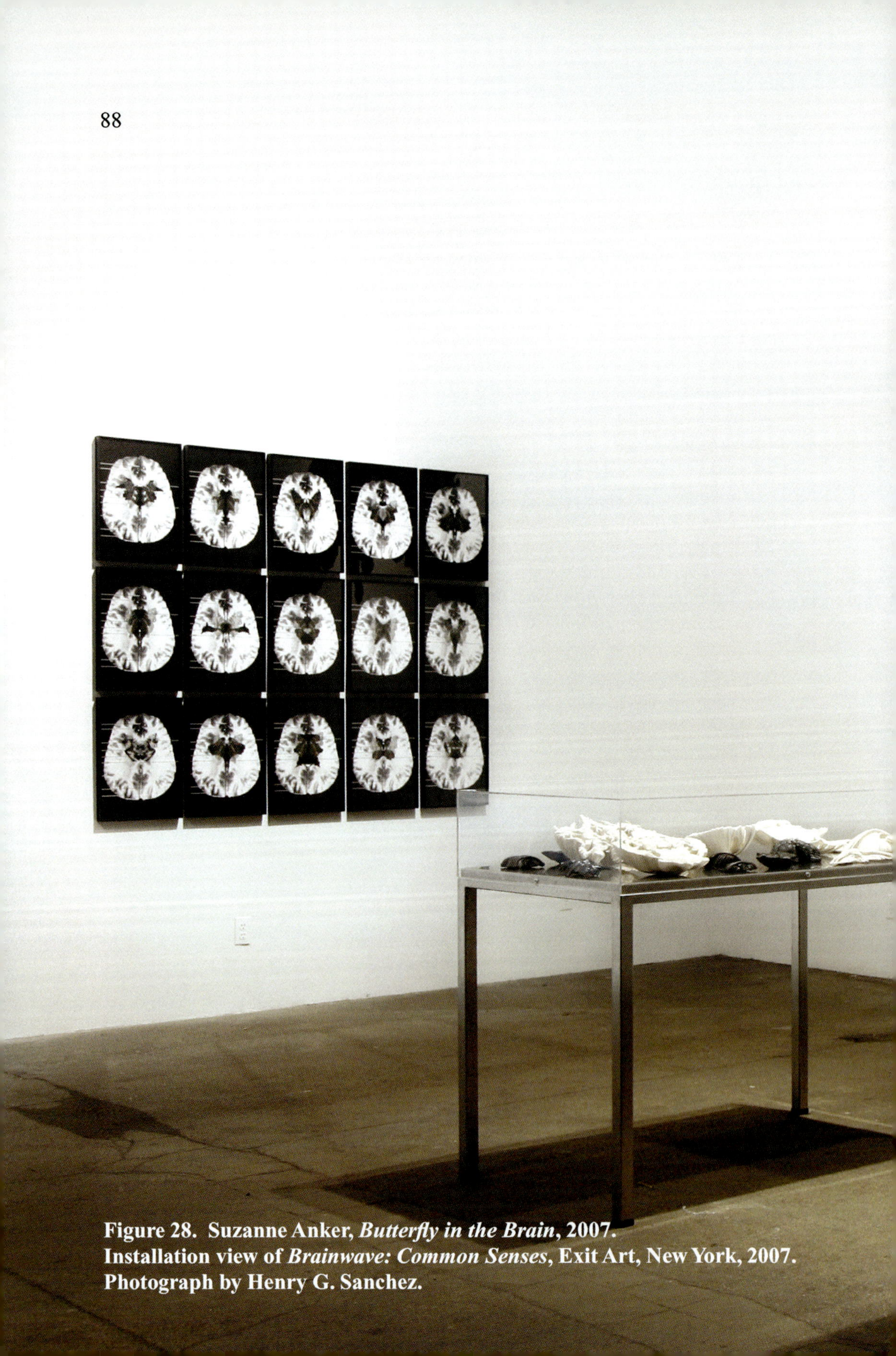

Figure 28. Suzanne Anker, *Butterfly in the Brain*, 2007. Installation view of *Brainwave: Common Senses*, Exit Art, New York, 2007. Photograph by Henry G. Sanchez.

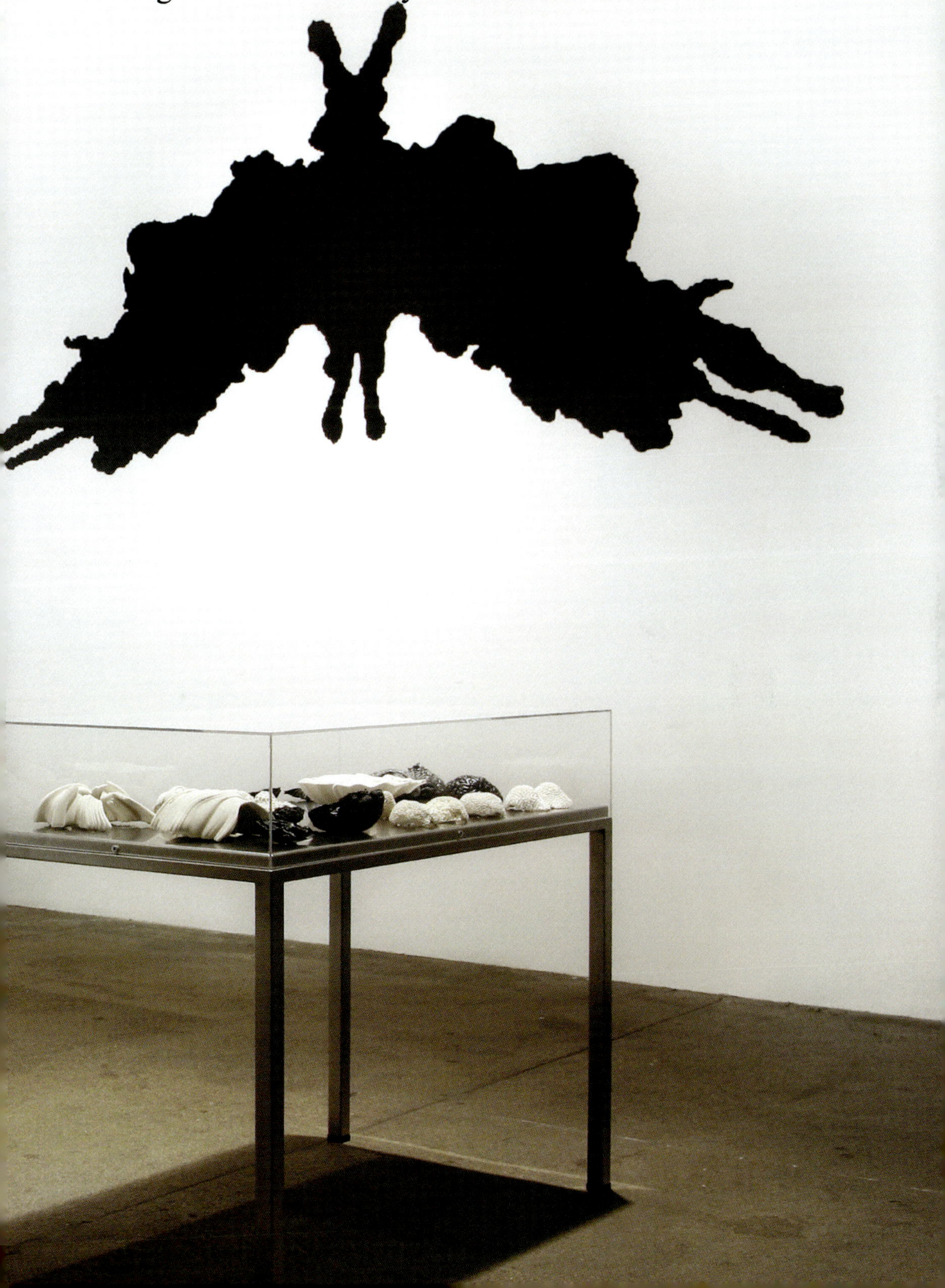

Dialogue II: The Butterfly in the Brain / Rorschach

SUZANNE ANKER & SABINE FLACH

Sabine Flach: *The Butterfly in the Brain* (2002) and *The Rorschach* series (2004) focused on the neurosciences as your subject matter. Why did this shift to the cognitive sciences replace your work with genetics?

Suzanne Anker: With the information revealed by the first draft of the Human Genome in 2000, various aspects of brain morphology, neurogenetic variation and gene expression, were being studied by scientists. New imaging technologies including fMRI, CAT scans and advanced sonograms revealed acute aspects of the workings of the human nervous system. The complexity of genetics and its variable permutations is certainly outdistanced by neurological processes. The neurosciences and their attendant landscapes also uncover and expand questions concerning perception, emotion, motion, cognition, and the unconscious. These sciences relate the workings of the brain to language acquisition and metaphorical structuring, as well as to bodily gestures. Thus, these concepts have an underscored affiliation with visual art practice. Questions concerning identity and memory are prominent components of many contemporary artists' work. Desires to picture thought and emotion have, especially since the invention of the X-ray, whetted the imagination of artists and lay people alike.[1]

SF: The installation *The Butterfly in the Brain* is a body of work consisting of objects, sculptures, charts and prints. Many were housed in plexiglass and stainless steel vitrines – a kind of museum display (fig. 28). On an adjoining wall a large-scale painted butterfly image is appropriated from Hermann Rorschach's original ink-blot test. All of these elements point to visualizing neuroscientific processes as employed by scientists. However, your work is in a form exempt from objectivity. What attributes of subjective experience are exposed through these images and objects?

SA: Unlike genetics, which is represented by discrete molecular entities, such as chromosomes, gene sequences, and symbolic letter forms, visualizing the neu-

1 See Linda Henderson, *Duchamp in Context: Science and Technology in the Large Glass and Related Works* (Princeton : Princeton University Press, 1998) and Bettyann Kevles, *Naked to the Bone Medical Imaging in the Twentieth Century* (New Brunswick, N.J.: Rutgers University Press, 1997).

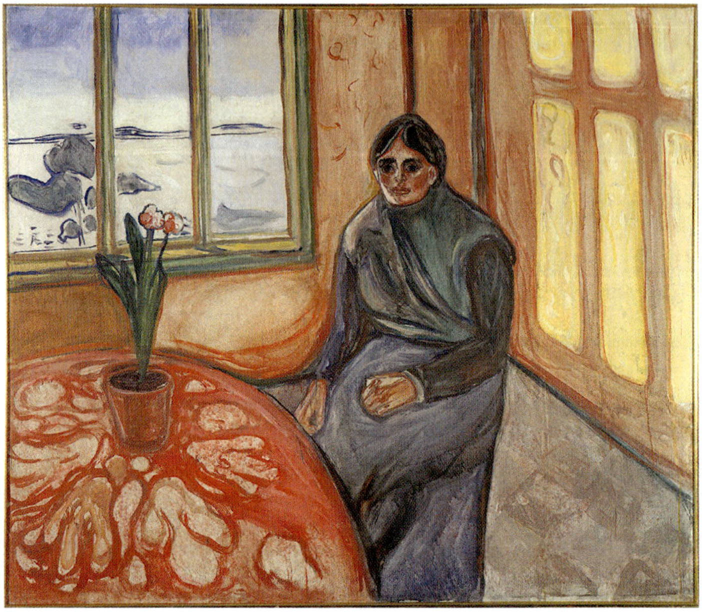

Figure 29. Edvard Munch: *Melankoli (Laura)*, 1899. Oil on Canvas, 43.3 x 49.6 in (110 x 126 cm) © The Munch Museum / The Munch-Ellingsen Group / Artists Rights Society (ARS), NY.

rosciences is more ephemeral. How can a brain in action be portrayed? What do dream images look like or mean? How are the emotions delineated? Since the brain functions as an organ in operation, how are its working aspects to be presented as visual images? This subject remains a significant idiom for artists to explore.

SF: Edvard Munch is most well known for his iconic work *The Scream* (1893) which expressed the anxiety accompanying the turn of the 19th century into the 20th. Many of his paintings dealt with psychological issues, such as *Melankoli (Laura)* (fig. 29), a portrait of his depressive sister. Munch's use of the brain as a pattern on a tablecloth is much more than a motif. It resonates with emerging theories of psychology and pathology of his time. How would you connect yourself to this motif in his work?

SA: During the 19th century, advances in the sciences were explicitly within the public domain. The French anatomist, physiologist and sculptor Paul Richer suggested that "art could renew itself by looking to science" with its modes of "observation, experimentation, analysis and hypotheses, which were equally appli-

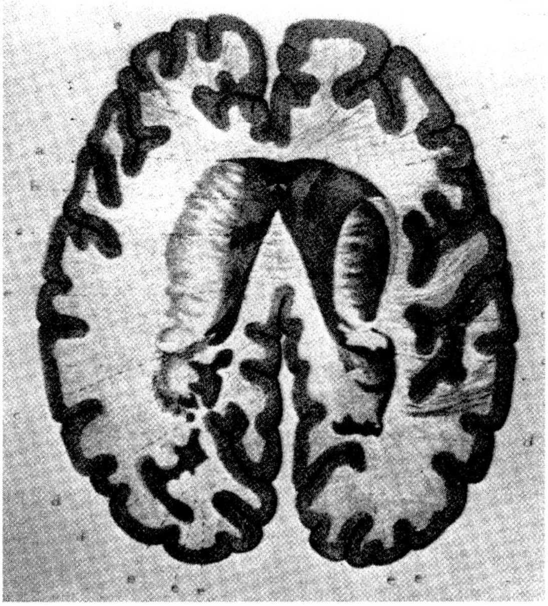

Figure 30. Jean-Martin Charcot. Horizontal sections *(s)* of the cerebrum, displaying the islets of sclerosis in different regions. Plate II from Jean-Martin Charcot, Lectures on the Diseases of the Nervous System (Academy of Medicine, 1962, Facsimile of the London print, 1881)
© New York Academy of Medicine.

cable to creative invention."[2] For Edvard Munch, whose father and brother were physicians, an awareness of the pictorial means for manifesting the physiology of the brain alongside emotional states of being became an aesthetic concern. The relationship between mind and body formed a discourse in psychophysiology, erupting as an attempt to find material causes for the emotions. Regarding *Melankoli (Laura),* the late Kirk Varnedoe suggested that the tablecloth in the lower left pictorially resembles brain tissue. He states that it is modeled "after the tinted coronal brain sections which were used to illustrate neurological abnormalities in contemporary medical publications. This neuroanatomical allusion functions as a specific exterior reference to Laura's internal condition." This painting, Varnedoe goes on, "reflects Munch's Symbolist concern with the materialization of invisible impulses, and with psychological, not representational, portraiture."[3]

2 Shelley Wood Cordulack, *Edvard Munch and the Physiology of Symbolism* (Madison, N.J.: Fairleigh Dickinson University Press, 2002).

3 Kirk Varnedoe, *Northern Light: Realism and Symbolism in Scandinavian Painting, 1880-1910* (Brooklyn, NY: Brooklyn Museum, 1982).

Another seminal figure in neuroscience is Jean-Martin Charcot (1825-1893). Although famous for his work on hysteria and hypnosis, he was also the first to diagnose many afflictions of the nervous system (fig. 30). Employing clinical observation as a tool to reveal physical symptoms attendant with anatomical dissection, Charcot diagnosed various neurological diseases such as multiple sclerosis (MS), amyotrophic lateral sclerosis (ALS) and a neuropathy called Charcot-Marie-Tooth disease. The developing investigation into organic and non-organic nervous disorders in the late 19th century encompassed depression, anxiety, phobias, seizures and tremors. Calling into question the relationship of mind and body, the exploration of the brain and its neural networks continues on this trajectory, enhanced by functional neuroimaging technologies permitting a glimpse of the brain in action. In the *MRI Butterfly* series an image of a butterfly is superimposed over an image of a Rorschach test, which is again layered on top of a generic image of a MRI brain scan (figs. 31-33). Set to music by Erik Satie, the compound images keep rhythm with the music in a stop-and-go dance, emitting the feeling of fleeting thoughts entering and exiting the mind.

Theories of mind and brain continue to operate in academic circles concerning the brain's cultural axis. There have been numerous exhibitions enveloping the neurosciences within visual art practice.[4] Moreover, Semir Zeki, a prominent neuroscientist at University College London in the United Kingdom, considers artists to be neuroscientists as well.[5] The problem with his approach is that Zeki does not discriminate between kinds of images and their visual histories. Neuroscientific images can be repurposed by moving them into the cultural domain where their status is altered. The most relevant of these images is my MRI Butterfly animation, which metaphorically shows the brain in action.

SF: Why did you choose brains, butterflies and chromosomes? What links them together?

SA: These early works employ nature's symmetry as bridges between brain morphology, butterfly patterns and microscopic images of chromosomes. In each case they become symbols of transfiguration. The human brain is divided into dual hemispheres where synaptic connectivity creates memory, language, and locomotion. The butterfly, originating as a crawling caterpillar, manifests an intrigu-

4 See Suzanne Anker, *Fundamentally Human: Contemporary Art and Neuroscience = Temelde İnsan: çağdaş sanat ve nörobilim*. ed. Begüm Akkoyunlu et al. (Tepebaşı, İstanbul: Pera Museum, 2011). Catalogue published in conjunction with an exhibition of the same title at the Pera Museum, in Istanbul, Turkey in April, 2011.

5 Semir Zeki is Professor of Neuroaesthetics at UCL. His books include: *A Vision of the Brain*; *Inner Vision* and *An Exploration of Art and the Brain*.

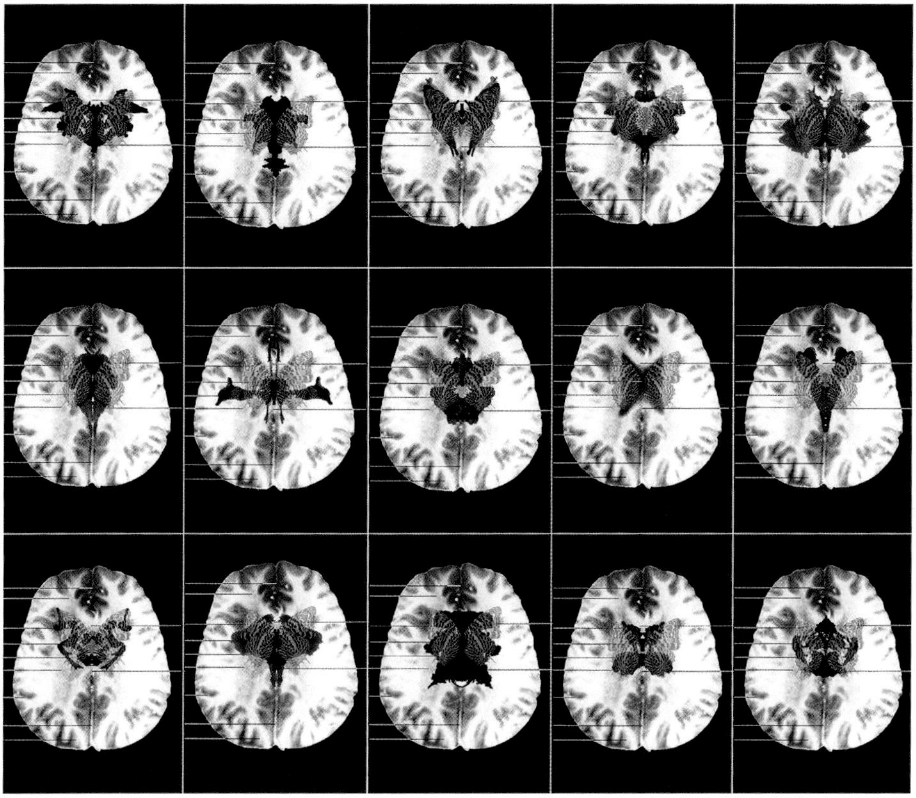

Figure 31. Suzanne Anker, *MRI Butterfly* series, 2008.
15 Archival inkjet prints on paper, 13 x 19 in (33 x 48.2 cm) each.

ing metamorphosis into a splendid winged creature. Similarly, the chromosome changes its form when it merges with another somatic cell to form a zygote, which in turn is regenerated as offspring.

SF: The title of the exhibition *The Butterfly in the Brain* is quite intriguing. How did you come to choose it?

SA: The title of the exhibition is a reframing of the common expression: "I have butterflies in my stomach." This condition, which I am sure everyone has felt at some point in their lives, is a burst of anxiety produced by hormonal reactions stimulated by circumstance. Examples include, speaking in front of a large audience, nervously waiting for your first date, or hearing that you have been nominated for an impressive award. Another aspect of this title substitutes the brain for the gut. A "second brain" is in the involuntary gut, in the intestines where the endemic nervous system resides and is charged with neuronal transmissions (fig. 34).

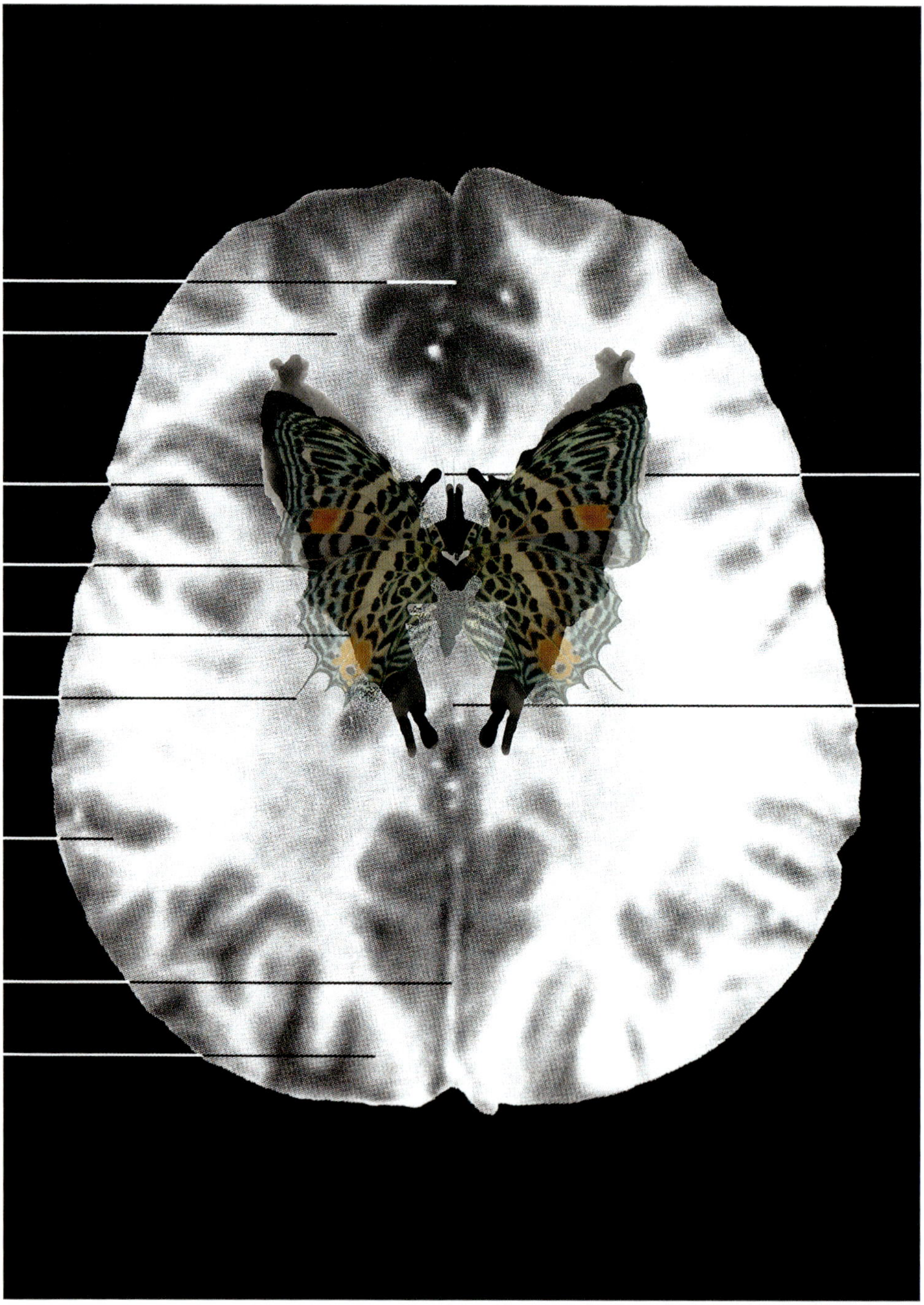

Figure 32. Suzanne Anker, *MRI Butterfly #3*, 2008.
Archival inkjet print on paper, 13 x 19 in (33 x 48.2 cm).

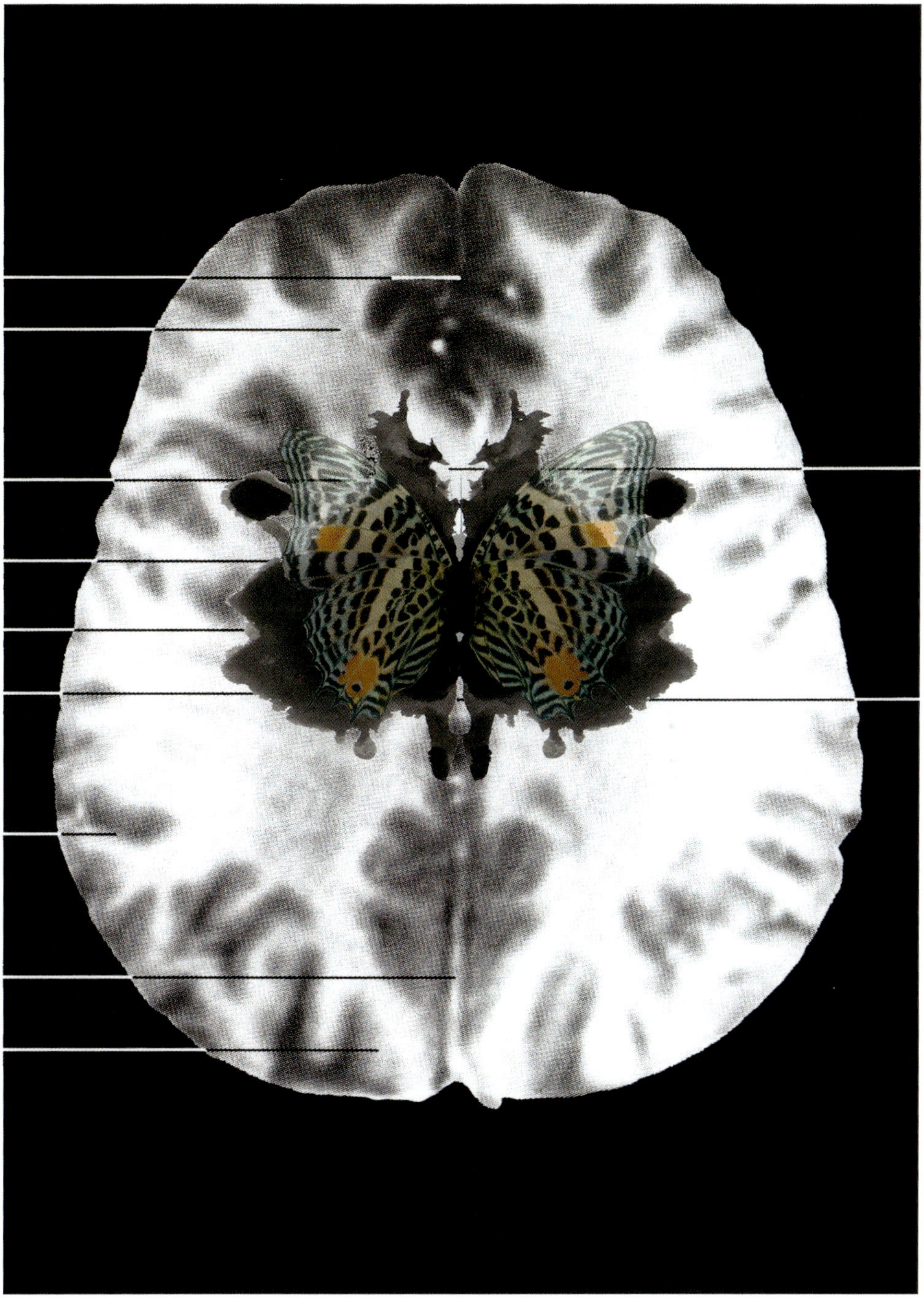

Figure 33. Suzanne Anker, *MRI Butterfly #5*, 2008.
Archival inkjet print on paper, 13 x 19 in (33 x 48.2 cm).

SF: For the neuro- and cognitive sciences image-making processes play a significant role. Your neuroscientifically-inspired projects function as interventions into image-producing processes. They are signifiers that point to the fact that we can't take these processes at face value, whether they are brain scans or projective tests. Please describe the relevance of these images for your work as opposed to their "scientific" utility.

SA: Images, like the nervous system itself, are highly complex entities. Their meaning and use is contextual and empirically based. Currently neuro-imagery such as fMRI represent, as I have stated, the brain in action in real time. The pictures are in fact reassembled from computer-generated numerical data sets that measure blood flow to the brain. Appearing as empirical information gathered through technology, they do point to neurological processes indirectly. Their status as data is sometimes contradictory, even unreliable. They are not iconic portraits of the brain's activity. They are translations that are set to computational thresholds. Recently there has been a lot of controversy regarding how to interpret such images. The understanding of the brain through its anatomy and morphology is now being amplified due to new imaging technologies, which encompass the picturing of neurons in action. The public at large has always been fascinated by the possibility of seeing someone's thoughts or reading one's mind. Some of the applications of this technology are, unfortunately, edging towards a neo-phrenology.[6] Possibilities for uncovering sub-rosa thoughts, predicting violence and other deviant behaviors are being bantered around by experts who see these tools as both dangerous and life affirming. The public has visited this scenario in film, where "pre-cogs" can predict crime in Hollywood's *Minority Report.* My work in this area brings these images out into a cultural domain, divorced from disease and interpretation, as symbols of current scientific imaging devices and their critical surround.

SF: I want to focus now on the *Rorschach* series. The *Rorschach* images are two-dimensional, their forms developing by coincidence in the process of their making. Could you describe the significance of these forms in your work?

SA: Although controversial at best, Rorschachs are psychological projective tests widely recognized by a public audience. To some extent they have become cultural icons. Appearing in the work of Andy Warhol and Annette Messager, among others, the Rorschach continues its occult status as a possible lens into the public imagination. Originating as a children's game called *Blotto,* inkblots are em-

6 Ed Diener, "Neuroimaging: Voodoo, New Phrenology, or Scientific Breakthrough? Introduction to Special Section on fMRI." *Perspectives on Psychological Science* 5, no. 6, 714-715.

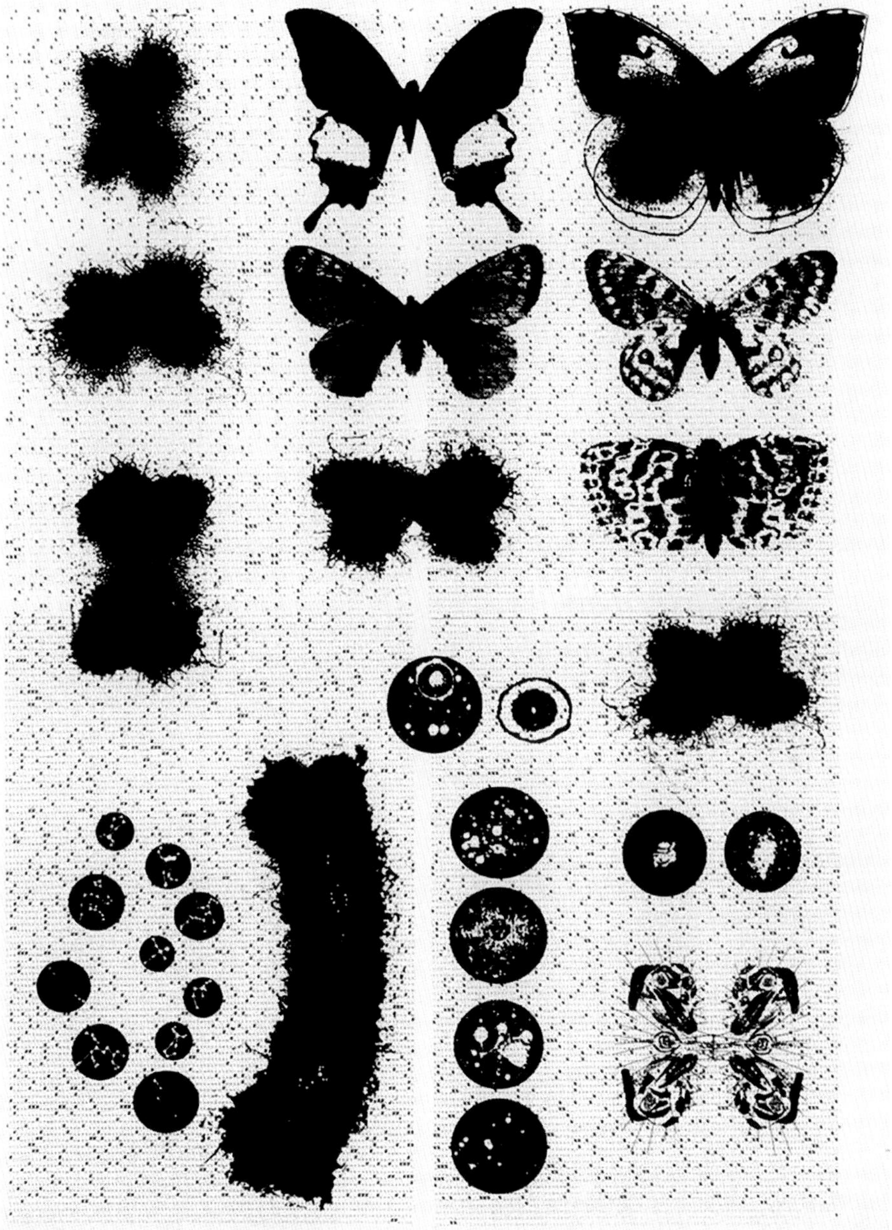

Figure 34. Suzanne Anker, *Papillon, 2002*. From the *Codex Eyespot* series. Silkscreen print on frosted mylar, 36 x 24 in (91.4 x 60.9 cm).

ployed as stimuli, intent on forcing the unconscious to turn over its quarry. The Rorschach has become a vernacular word, a kind of opinion poll expression, a cultural icon[7] (figs. 35-37).

Historian of science Peter Galison describes the Rorschach test in the following way: "In a brown cardboard box comes ten cards, printed in Bern Switzerland. The publisher Verlag Hans Huber is so concerned about the quality of their reproduction that it will only use the same antique printing presses that stamped out the first edition in 1921. And it won't print at all if the humidity and temperature do not match the secret instructions that have been passed down over generations. At the same time this box of plates may well be the most studied object of the last hundred years: several million people have not only examined them but recorded the innermost details of what they saw. What are these cards? To answer (or even not to answer) is to present yourself."[8]

As symmetrical structures of random forms, my specific interest in the Rorschach tests are based on their conversion into sculptural objects. Using the three-dimensional modeling software Maya, the inkblot itself is turned into numerical code. Numbers turn into 3D forms, and 3D forms becomes decipherable as numerical code. Looking like bones, archaic sea creatures, body parts, etc., they become surrogates for the imagination itself, opening up dialogues between mind and body. In these works the mind is, literally, embodied. These sculptural forms are computer-generated objects, constructed one layer at a time much the way a sedimentary rock comes into existence through the deposition of silt.

7 Naamah Akavia, *Subjectivity in Motion: Life, Art, and Movement in the Work of Hermann Rorschach* (New York: Brunner-Routledge, 2013).

8 Peter Galison, "Image of Self." In *Things That Talk: Object Lessons from Art and Science*, ed Lorraine Daston (New York: Zone Books, 2007).

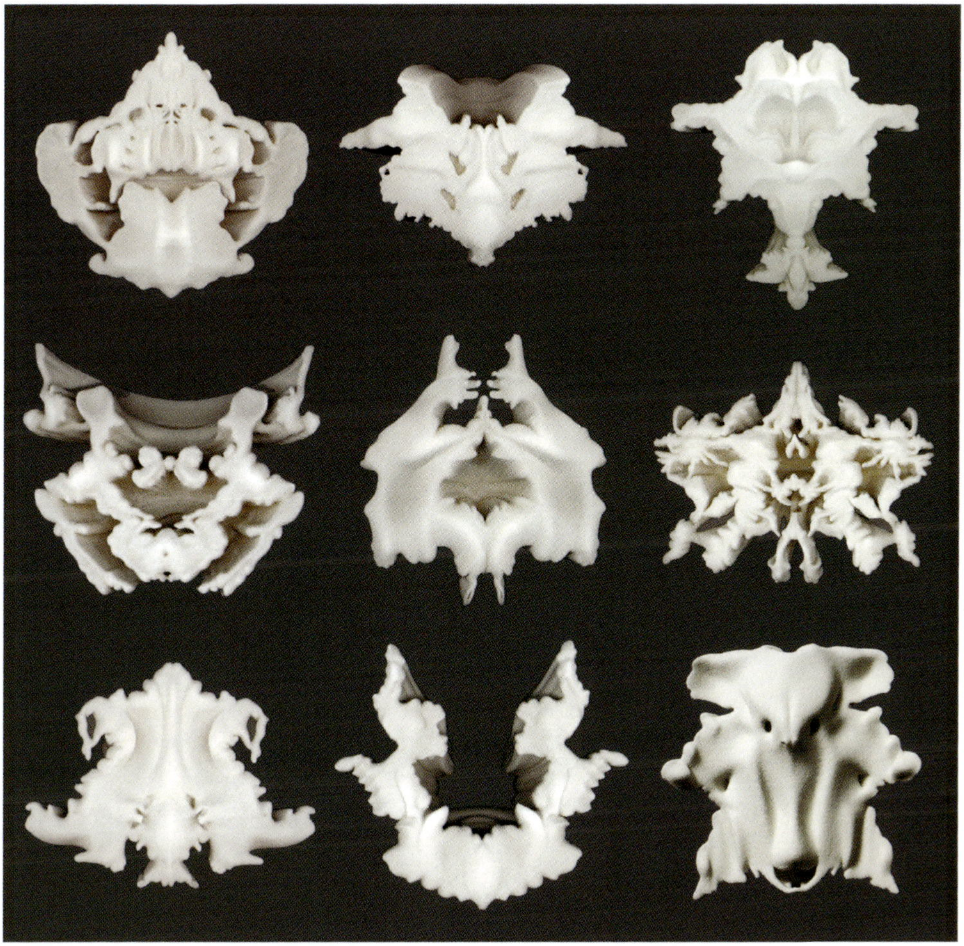

Figure 35. Six works from the *Rorschach* series by Suzanne Anker, 2004-05. Rapid prototype sculpture of plaster and resin, 4.5 x 4.5 x 2 in (11.4 x 11.4 x 5 cm) each. Top left: *Crab*; top center: *Wolf*; top right: *Tarantula*; middle left: *Gossipers*; middle center: *Cauldron*; middle right: *Spider*; bottom left: *Father*; bottom center: *Rocker*; bottom right: *Bear*.

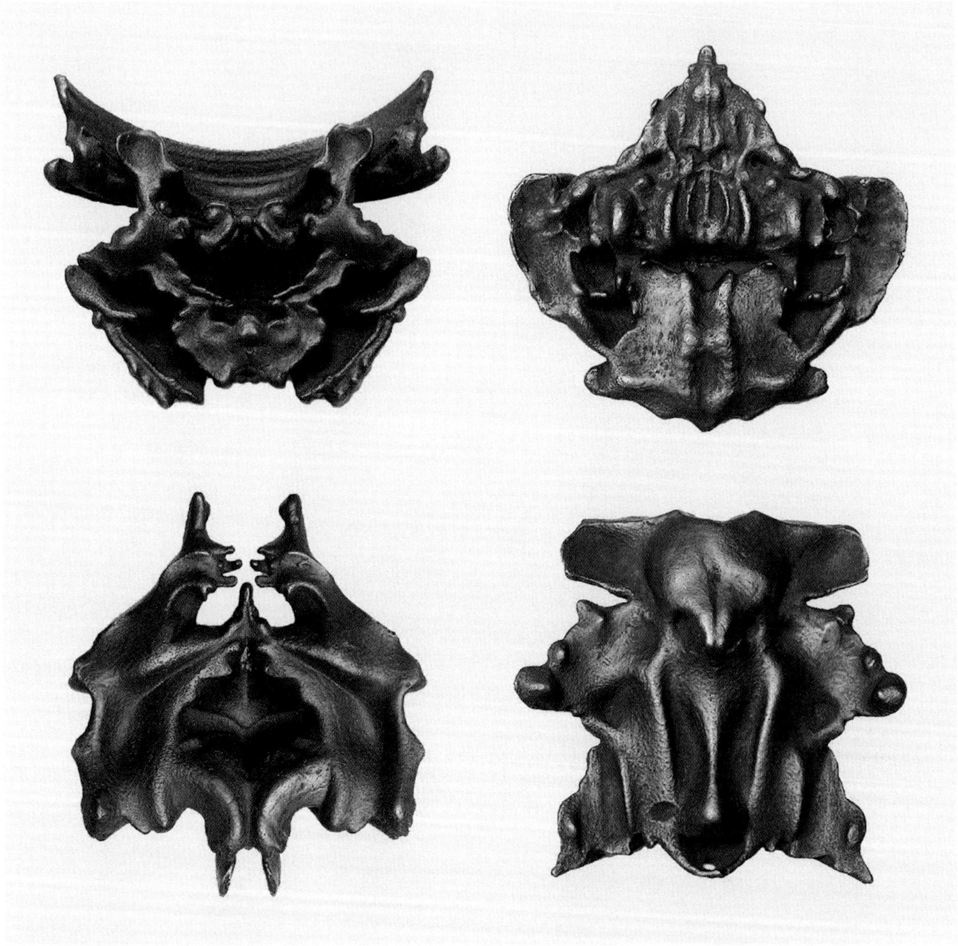

Figure 36. Front views of four works from the *Rorschach* series by Suzanne Anker, 2004-05. Cast bronze, 4.5 x 4.5 x 2 in (11.4 x 11.4 x 5 cm) each; Top left: *Gossipers*; Top right: *Crab*; Bottom left: *Cauldron*; Bottom right: *Bear*.

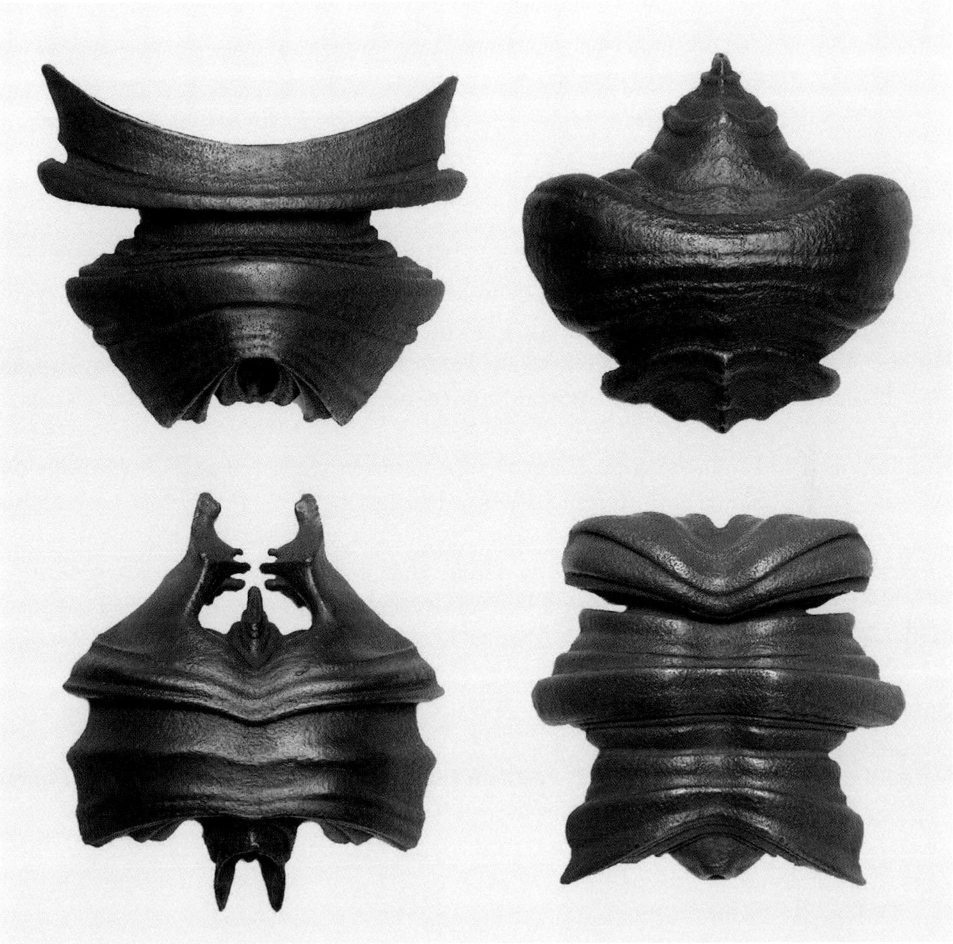

Figure 37. Back views of four works from the *Rorschach* series by Suzanne Anker, 2004-05. Cast bronze, 4.5 x 4.5 x 2 in (11.4 x 11.4 x 5 cm) each; Top left: *Gossipers*; Top right: *Crab*; Bottom left: *Cauldron*; Bottom right: *Bear*.

References

Akavia, Naamah. *Subjectivity in Motion: Life, Art, and Movement in the Work of Hermann Rorschach*. New York: Brunner-Routledge, 2013.

Anker, Suzanne. *Temelde İnsan: çağdaş sanat ve nörobilim = Fundamentally Human : Contemporary Art and Neuroscience*. Edited by Begüm Akkoyunlu and Tania Bahar. Tepeba ı, İstanbul: Pera Museum, 2011.

Cordulack, Shelley Wood. Edvard Munch and the Physiology of Symbolism. Madison [N.J.]: Fairleigh Dickinson University Press, 2002.

Diener, Ed. "Neuroimaging: Voodoo, New Phrenology, or Scientific Breakthrough? Introduction to Special Section on fMRI." *Perspectives on Psychological Science* 5, no. 6, 714-715.

Henderson, Linda Dalrymple. *Duchamp in Context: Science and Technology in the Large Glass and Related Works*. Princeton, N.J.: Princeton University Press, 1998.

Kevles, Bettyann. *Naked to the Bone Medical Imaging in the Twentieth Century*. New Brunswick, N.J.: Rutgers University Press, 1997.

Galison, Peter. "Image of Self." In *Things That Talk: Object Lessons from Art and Science*, edited by Lorraine Daston. New York: Zone Books, 2007.

Spielberg, Steven. *Minority Report*. 2002. Los Angeles, CA: 20th Century Fox, Film.

Varnedoe, Kirk. *Northern Light: Realism and Symbolism in Scandinavian Painting, 1880-1910*. Brooklyn, NY: Brooklyn Museum, 1982.

Zeki, Semir. *A Vision of the Brain*. Oxford: Blackwell Scientific Publications, 1993.

Zeki, Semir. *Inner Vision: An Exploration of Art and the Brain*. Oxford: Oxford University Press, 1999.

List of Illustrations

Fig. 28: Suzanne Anker, *Butterfly in the Brain*, 2007. Installation view of *Brain-Wave: Common Senses*, Exit Art, New York, 2007. Photograph by Herny G. Sanchez. Courtesy of Exit Art and the artist.
Fig. 29: Edvard Munch: *Melankoli (Laura)*, 1899. Oil on Canvas, 43.3 x 49.6 in (110 x 126 cm) © The Munch Museum / The Munch-Ellingsen Group / Artists Rights Society (ARS), NY.
Fig. 30: Jean-Martin Charcot. Horizontal sections *(s)* of the cerebrum, displaying the islets of sclerosis in different regions. Plate II from Jean-Martin Charcot, Lectures on the Diseases of the Nervous System (Academy of Medicine, 1962, Facsimile of the London print, 1881) © New York Academy of Medicine.
Fig. 31: Suzanne Anker, *MRI Butterfly* series, 2008. 15 Archival inkjet prints on paper, 13 x 19 in (33 x 48.2 cm) each.
Fig. 32: Suzanne Anker, *MRI Butterfly #3*, 2008. Archival inkjet print on paper, 13 x 19 in (33 x 48.2 cm).
Fig. 33: Suzanne Anker, *MRI Butterfly #5*, 2008. Archival inkjet print on paper, 13 x 19 in (33 x 48.2 cm).
Fig. 34: Suzanne Anker, *Papillon, 2002*. From the *Codex Eyespot* series. Silk-screen print on frosted mylar, 36 x 24 in (91.4 x 60.9 cm).
Fig. 35: Six works from the *Rorschach* series by Suzanne Anker, 2004-05. Rapid prototype sculpture of plaster and resin, 4.5 x 4.5 x 2 in (11.4 x 11.4 x 5 cm) each. Top left: *Crab*; top center: *Wolf*; top right: *Tarantula*; middle left: *Gossipers*; middle center: *Cauldron*; middle right: *Spider*; bottom left: *Father*; bottom center: *Rocker*; bottom right: *Bear*.
Fig. 36: Front views of four works from the *Rorschach* series by Suzanne Anker, 2004-05. Cast bronze, 4.5 x 4.5 x 2 in (11.4 x 11.4 x 5 cm) each; Top left: *Gossipers*; Top right: *Crab*; Bottom left: *Cauldron*; Bottom right: *Bear*.
Fig. 37: Back views of four works from the *Rorschach* series by Suzanne Anker, 2004-05. Cast bronze, 4.5 x 4.5 x 2 in (11.4 x 11.4 x 5 cm) each; Top left: *Gossipers*; Top right: *Crab*; Bottom left: *Cauldron*; Bottom right: *Bear*.

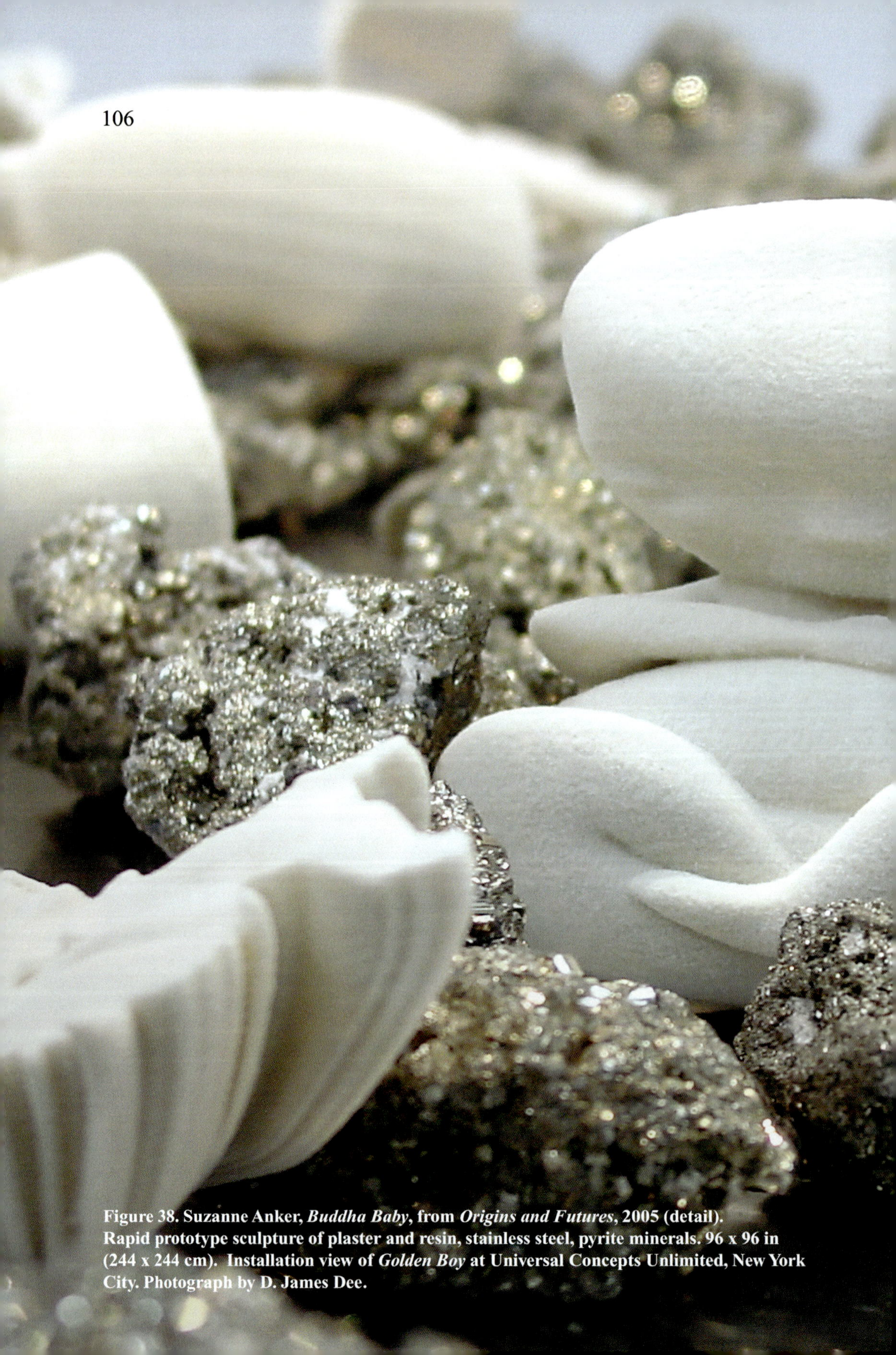

Figure 38. Suzanne Anker, *Buddha Baby*, from *Origins and Futures*, 2005 (detail). Rapid prototype sculpture of plaster and resin, stainless steel, pyrite minerals. 96 x 96 in (244 x 244 cm). Installation view of *Golden Boy* at Universal Concepts Unlimited, New York City. Photograph by D. James Dee.

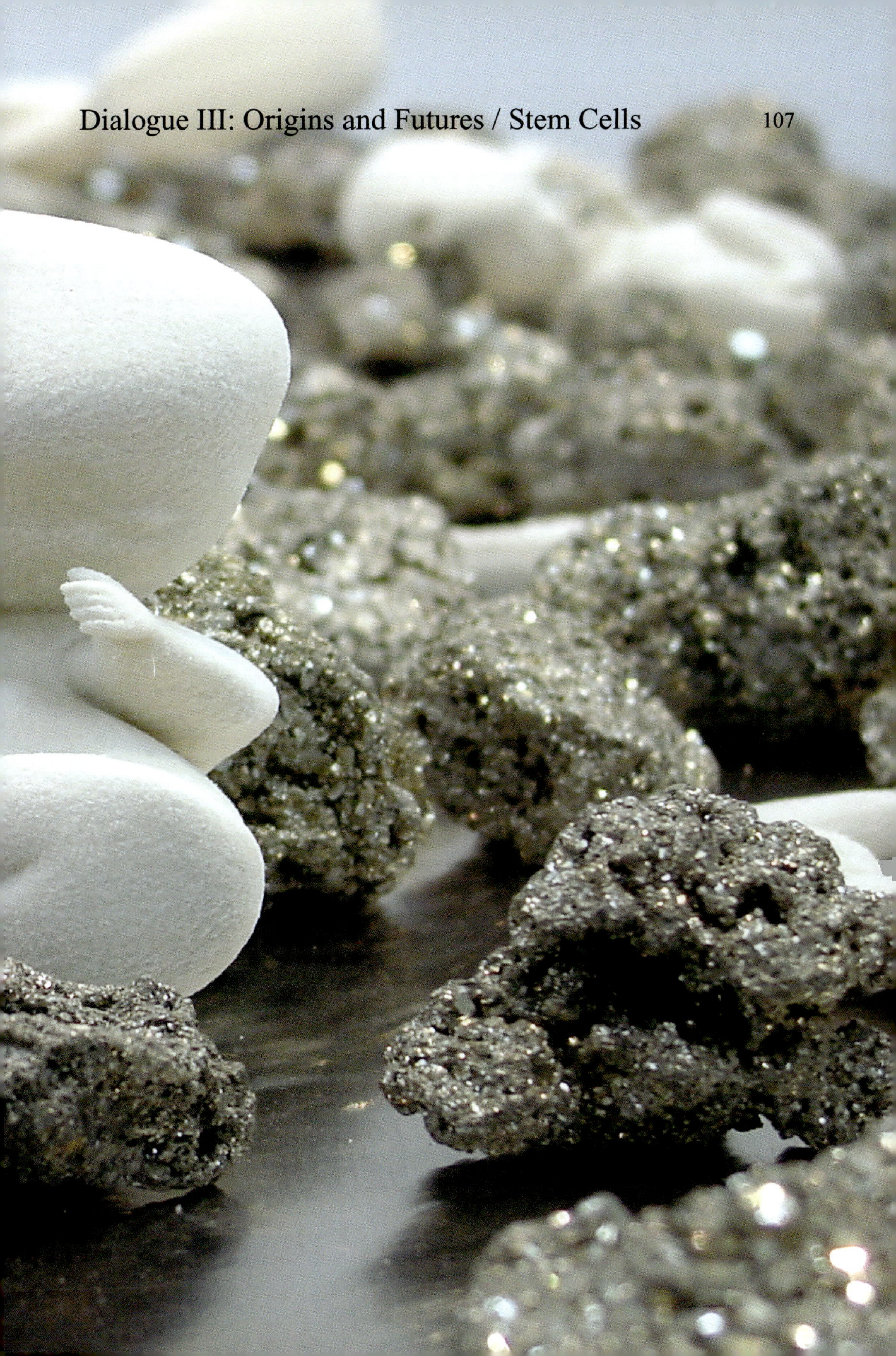

Dialogue III: Origins and Futures / Stem Cells

SUZANNE ANKER & SABINE FLACH

Sabine Flach: What relationship do you think exists between the biological sciences and the physical ones? During the 20th century, physics in particular, was the reigning paradigmatic science. In the 21st century, it is biology. How do you account for that shift?

Suzanne Anker: During the 20th century, biology was considered a "soft" science since it did not conform in exact ways to the underlying mathematical absolutism of space and time, gravity, relativity theory and the like. However, metaphors inherent in the physical sciences dominated the first half of the 20th century as in the art movements of Impressionism, Cubism, and Futurism, among others. These artistic developments incorporated uncertainty and flux influencing our perception and understanding of the physical world. Furthermore, highlighted by the discovery of X-rays by Wilhelm Röntgen in 1895, an invisible interior world was visualized for the first time, as this imaging device could render the body transparent.

With Watson and Crick's discovery of the structure of DNA in 1953, the image of the iconic atom was displaced by the double helix. Furthermore it was discovered that this charismatic molecule was responsible for the hereditary changes that passed on to future generations. As more allied technologies were invented and adapted to pursue this line of investigation, a molecular revolution was on its way. Genes, bits and particles could be isolated, mapped, transferred to other species and even patented. There are many examples of this narrative in *The Molecular Gaze*: *Art in the Genetic Age*, which I co-authored with the late sociologist of science, Dorothy Nelkin in 2003. The text remains an early platform on this subject linking art history with contemporary art and science studies.

SF: While the origins of life are still a mystery, we do realize that "life itself" is being transformed in the laboratory. What interest do you have in this regard? How can these concerns be visualized in art practice?

SA: When invoking origins, to what ancient evidence do we submit? Do we reference the primordial time when stardust fell to earth or when the first strings of living molecules replicated? Where did this marvelous journey of life begin? Such speculative questions remain unanswered, but continue to entice our imaginations. In 2003, I exhibited *Cyberchrome Chromosome (Hippopotamus)*, a sculpture that was catalogued as a standard form of karyotype. Karyotypes are charts of chromosomes, arranged by size and coordinated in numerical order.

These linear sequences discern the underlying structure of living matter and encode for differences concerning species and gender.

Cyberchrome Chromosome (Hippopotamus) was constructed from stainless steel wool, but one chromosome was fabricated from bronze wool, making it visually evident it was unlike the rest of the set. As a comment on the insertion of foreign genes, or even synthetic ones into already natural genomes, this work is a visualization of what future experiments might bring, at least on a genotypic level. This exhibit was held in conjunction with the 50th anniversary celebration of the discovery of the structure of DNA, at the New York Academy of Sciences.[1] In her review of the exhibitions, New York Times' critic Sarah Boxer described the piece as "witty and bright," but expressed dismay over many artists' moralizing about genetic engineering.[2]

SF: Please talk about *Origins and Futures*, a sculptural installation bringing together objects from the natural world alongside fabricated ones.

SA: In *Origins and Futures* (figs. 38-40), pyrite, a mineral commonly known as "fool's gold" glimmers with novelty and seduction. Its crystalline structure and reflecting light attracts the viewer's eye without hesitation. The piece is based on A.G. Cairns-Smith's hypothesis that primitive RNA learned to duplicate itself by taking over the crystalline lattice of a mineral, of which pyrite is an example.[3] After appropriating the crystal's structure, duplication processes were learned, thus leading to DNA's replication powers. That is one theory among many competing ones concerning the origin of life. However, in a commodity-driven economy, what parameters determine the future of life? Genes and their sequences are currently being patented by corporations, although such materials had never before been slated as intellectual property. This state of affairs provokes the entangled question as to whether our origins and futures are up for sale? And at what fair price do we assume that nature is a fungible commodity? By what means can these molecular entities be traded as financial instruments? Will they end up in a financial portfolio of derivatives? Futures are a speculative form of investment in money market offerings, while human genes have also come to be regarded as a form of bio-ore in this 21st century landscape.

1 It was one of many participating institutions in New York City, including the International Center of Photography (ICP), and The Graduate Center, City University of New York (CUNY). At the New York Academy of Sciences, Dorothy Nelkin and I curated *From Code to Commodity: Genetics and Visual Art*, an exhibition of work including Kate Storey, Kevin Clarke and the late Frank Moore among others.

2 Sarah Boxer, "At Play With DNA," *The New York Times*, March 14, 2003, 35-39.

3 A. G. Cairns-Smith, *Seven Clues to the Origin of Life: A Scientific Detective Story* (Cambridge: Cambridge University Press, 1990).

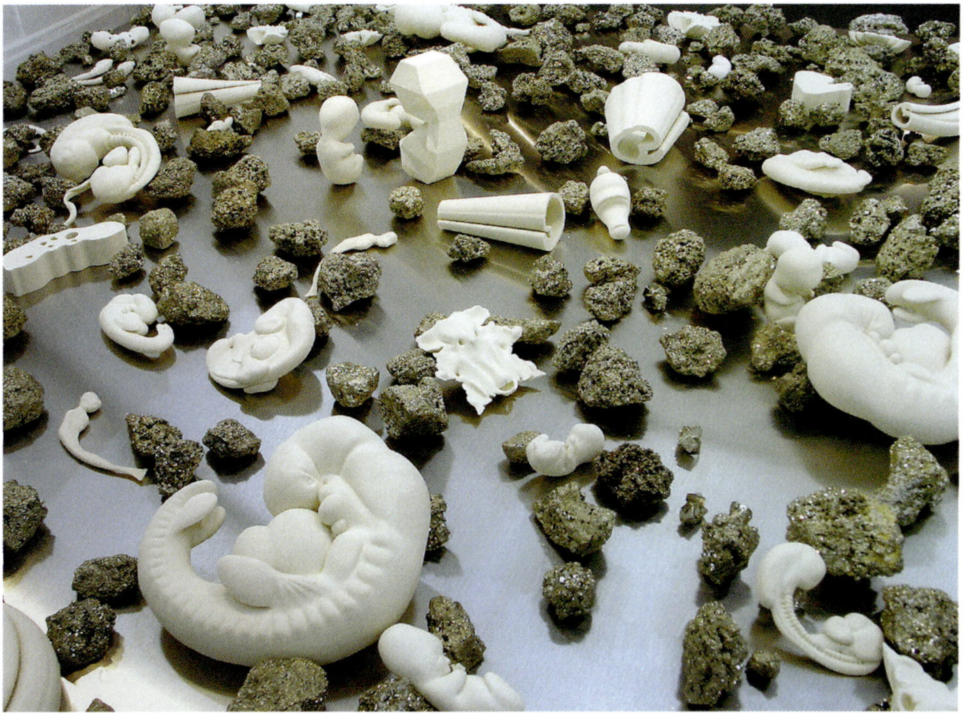

Figure 39. Suzanne Anker, *Origins and Futures*, 2005 (detail). Rapid prototype sculpture of plaster and resin, stainless steel, pyrite minerals, 96 x 96 in (244 x 244 cm). Installation view of *Golden Boy* at Universal Concepts Unlimited, New York City. Photograph by D. James Dee.

SF: Gene sequences are being commodified even when they do not point to underlying causes of disease. Where do you think lines should be drawn in this regard?

SA: There has been much controversy over this issue. The simple fact is that I don't own my personally given DNA. And neither do you. I find this quite troubling. Since I have not extracted and decoded its underlying molecular structure, I do not qualify for a patent on my own hereditary material. Patents have traditionally been given to inventions, but more recently patents can be obtained for synthetic chemical markers, tissue and cellular samples, genetically modified organisms and the like. Although there are differences between life forms and their subcellular levels as opposed to mechanic devices and tools, industry in cooperation with policy officials are granting such applications as an attempt to jump start new businesses and products.

SF: As biomaterials become products for sale, how does this concept relate to earlier attitudes toward the industrialization of science itself?

SA: After World War II and the onset of the Cold War the term "Big Science" was coined. At this time in American history, a myriad of war technologies became instrumental vehicles for the expansion of science and medicine. The sphere of science projects included large-scale ventures requiring funding from the government and allied corporations. This enterprise was referred to by the notable United States President Dwight D. Eisenhower as the "military-industrial complex." It is within this framework that Big Science exists today. Laurie Anderson's debut album with Warner Brothers in 1982 entitled *Big Science* was both a tribute to technology and a warning about its apocalyptic role in society. Anderson, a regular figure in the downtown art world, had recently turned away from strictly visual art to concentrate on integrating synthetic sound into her work.

SF: Alongside Anderson, the term *surrogacy* also emerged in the 80s. This term has a double meaning, could you please explain?

SA: American artist Allan McCollum began referring to his artworks in the late 70s as "plaster surrogates." His pieces, appearing as Minimalist paintings and organized in salon-style serialized objects, were intended to be stand-ins or proxys for paintings. Functioning as emblems for the ironically artificial, they are composed of cast plaster and painted black. The pieces pointed towards the reproductive and repetitive needs of a never-ending consumer-driven mass culture in the same era that saw the birth of surrogate motherhood, a substitutive method of gestation. Employed as a night janitor in an office building in downtown Manhattan, McCollum would gaze into the empty offices across streets evocative of desolate canyons. He talks about the circumstances behind his *Surrogate Paintings* as the result of his opportunity to look into the office spaces housed in other buildings across the way and see paintings hanging on the walls. Although he couldn't quite make out their content he began thinking of such paintings as anonymous objects that functioned primarily to fill wall space. He went on to construct an object symbolizing a painting. He included a framing device, a traditional mat and a monochromatic field inside.

Casting this iconic recipe in hydrostone and then painting the internal surfaces of the objects with black enamel, the artist arranged the pictures as gallery installations in a 19th century salon-style. Grouped as sets of small, repetitive squares and rectangles, McCollum's *Surrogate Paintings* have a decidedly cool air about them, satirizing painting as a fetish-commodity. Also revealing an ironic twist concentrated in ideas of abstract painting and Minimalism, this gesture initiated considerations about specialized objects such as "art" and what they stand for in a mass-mediated culture. As surface veneer representing as closely as possible the object of desire, a surrogate is a stand-in or substitute.

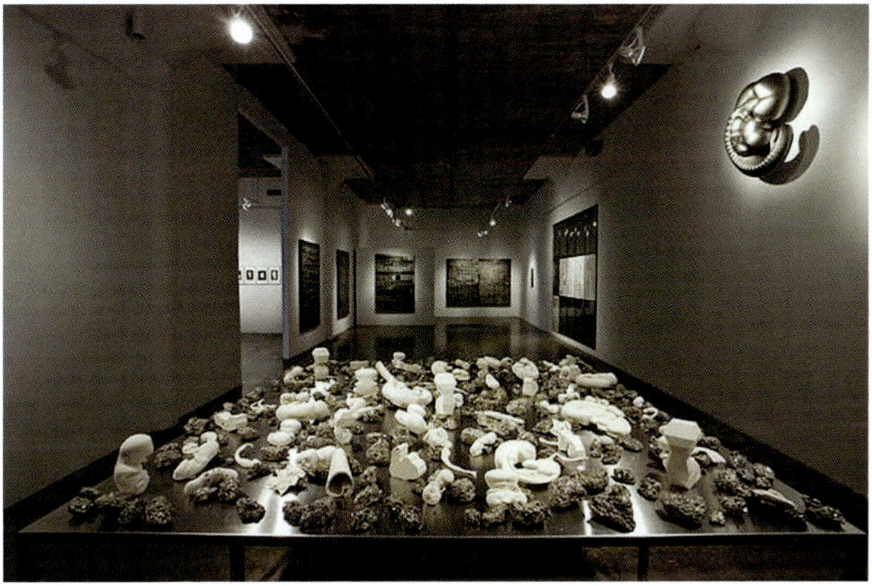

Figure 40. Suzanne Anker, *Origins and Futures*, 2005. Rapid prototype sculpture of plaster and resin, stainless steel, pyrite minerals, 96 x 96 in (244 x 244 cm). Installation view of *FutureNatural* at Deborah Colton Gallery, Houston, Texas.

Is a substitute, a surrogate, or a look-alike yet another form of art historian George Kubler's replications? Can we conceive of the McCollum surrogates as a debased form of Minimalism or the beginning of a pattern that changes direction? As a cultural meme, surrogacy has leaked into cultural and social norms far removed from Minimalism's Gestalt aesthetic. Do we view surrogate motherhood as a degraded form of motherhood, or, on the other hand, has it become an opportunity for reconfiguring traditional beliefs? How shall such patterns of imitation be viewed in art, culture, and the social world?

In 1980 the first contract for surrogate motherhood was legally adopted in the United States – surrogacy became a technique for "womb renting." Unlike hotels or motels, where the terms "vacancy" or "no vacancy" can be employed to denote full or empty, wombs are not empty spaces. During the process of gestation, blood flows graciously from mother to child. The amniotic fluid in which the unborn swims is littered with the birth mother's cells and may, in addition, contain cellular matter from earlier offspring. Generally women who act as surrogates are in need of financial remuneration, especially in Mexico and India. Left with few resources to provide better lives for their families they engage in this procedure. There are also many brokers, lawyers and middlemen who arrange such agreements. It is now possible for a couple's zygote to be cryogenetically delivered to a far-off land and inserted into a surrogate's womb. I find some similarities here with the contractual agreements for mail-order brides and wet nurses in the 19th century. In each scenario, "working-class bodies" are employed to support middle- to upper-class desires.

SF: You cited the working class body – let's focus on that for a moment. One of the most significant changes in traditional motifs related to the representation of women is the Venus. Édouard Manet shocked the art world in 1863 by transforming Titian's *Venus of Urbino* and Giorgione's *Sleeping Venus* into what has become his scandalous *Olympia*. In his work, Olympia looks directly towards the viewer, eye to eye. Uncommon for models in the 19th century to appear with such an aggressive gaze, the artist portrays her as a subject in control, even as more details identify her as a prostitute. How do these motifs relate to the status of women today?

SA: What connects the role of women in society today to an earlier time is the consideration of women as object. Cultural studies have addressed the notions of race, class and gender for several decades. However these issues continue to resurface in alternative ways. The surrogate mother is an example, as well as young women and men who sell their gametes or even placentas. Frequently in India and other third-world nations, although illegal, kidneys and bones go to the highest bidder. The body as a site of commerce is certainly being revisited by new reproductive technologies and transplantation procedures. From prostitution to migrant workers to the exploitation of low-wage foreign workers, what discourses beyond Karl Marx can be formulated to reconcile these issues in the 21st century? Even in Edgard Degas' *At The Races* (1869), a paid wet nurse breast feeds the infant, while the mother – and others – look on. Is a body just a commodity, a thing that can be purchased for labor or parts?

There has been an exponential rise in the number of available surrogates as gay couples and bereaved families desire or are in need of genetically related offspring. 21st-century technologies have allowed for the creation of "savior siblings," which entails bringing a child into the world so that it could be a genetic match for a very ill sibling.

Surrogacy is a term that not only refers to pregnancy or appropriation, but also has embedded aspects of imitation and the artificial – cultural issues in the forefront of post-industrial societies. These are vanguard questions on the leading edge of bioethics, where corpses can become fathers, children can be the offspring of more than on set of parents, and gametes can be harvested and sold to the highest bidder.

SF: Your exhibition in 2004 entitled *Golden Boy* consisted of large scale digital

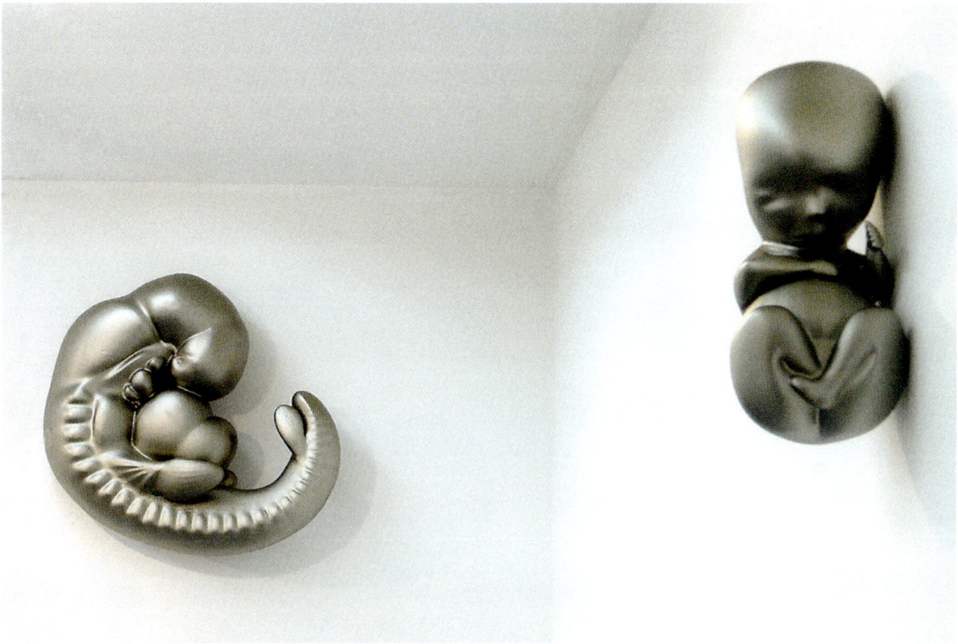

Figure 41. Left: Suzanne Anker, *First Fetus*, 2004. Rapid prototype sculpture, urethane foam and acrylic, 25 x 38 x 13 in (63.5 x 96.5 x 33 cm). Right: Suzanne Anker, *Golden Boy*, 2004. Rapid prototype sculpture, urethane foam and acrylic, 16 x 24 x 18 in (40.6 x 61 x 45.7 cm).

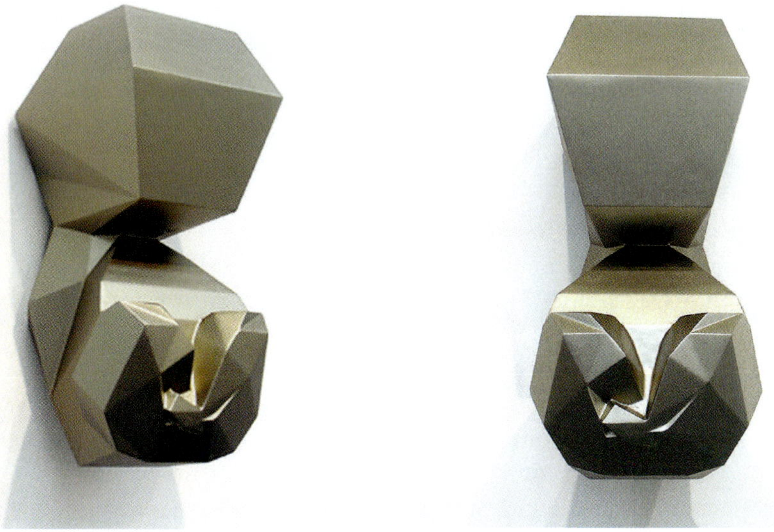

Figure 42. Suzanne Anker, *Cubist Baby*, 2004. Rapid prototype sculpture, urethane foam and acrylic. 32 x 16 x 16 in (81 x 40 x 40 cm).

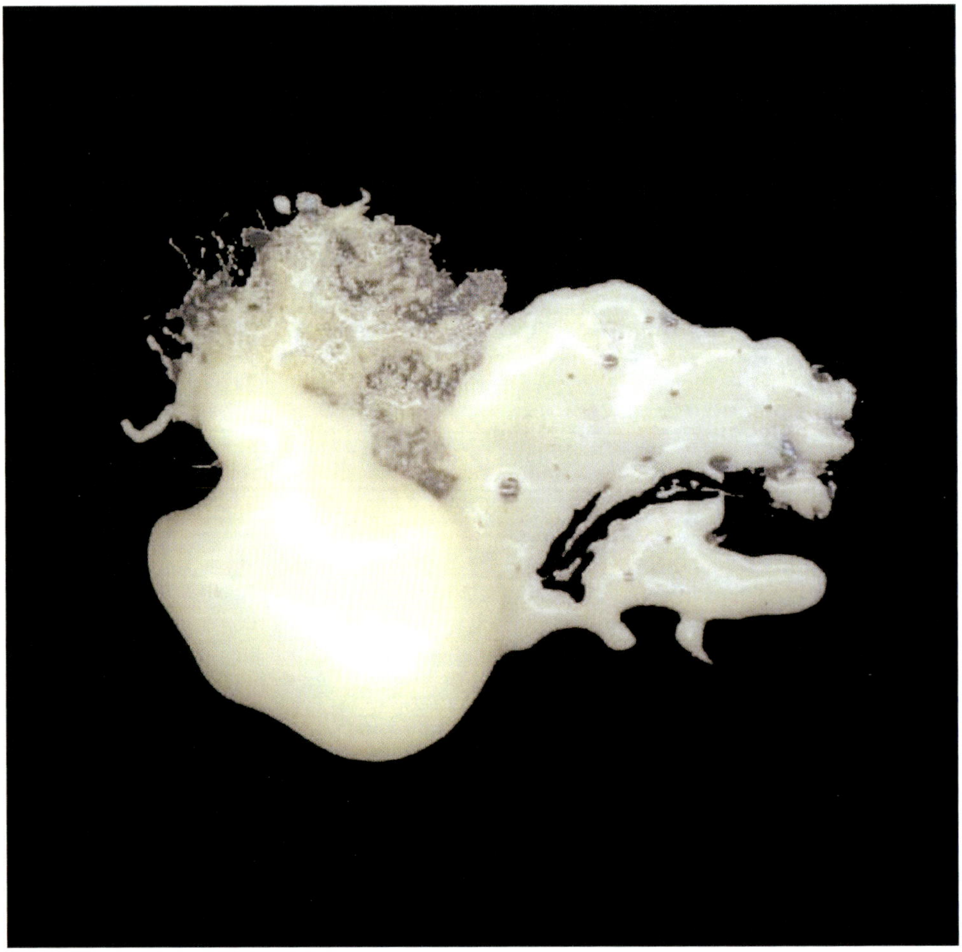

Figure 43. Suzanne Anker, *Stem Cells #4*, 2004.
Archival inkjet print on paper, 13 x 19 in (33 x 48 cm).

sculpture hung on the wall as well as a stainless steel table covered with pyrite and plaster and resin "fetuses" in varying degrees of maturity. Why did you title the exhibition *Golden Boy*?

SA: Worldwide there is a preference among would-be parents for a male child. With new imaging and reproductive technologies at hand it is now possible to ascertain the gender of your offspring before it is born. In some countries, where sonograms are inexpensive and abortions legal, a great many female fetuses have been aborted. These personal actions have created an imbalance between the number of females born in relation to the number of males in these countries.

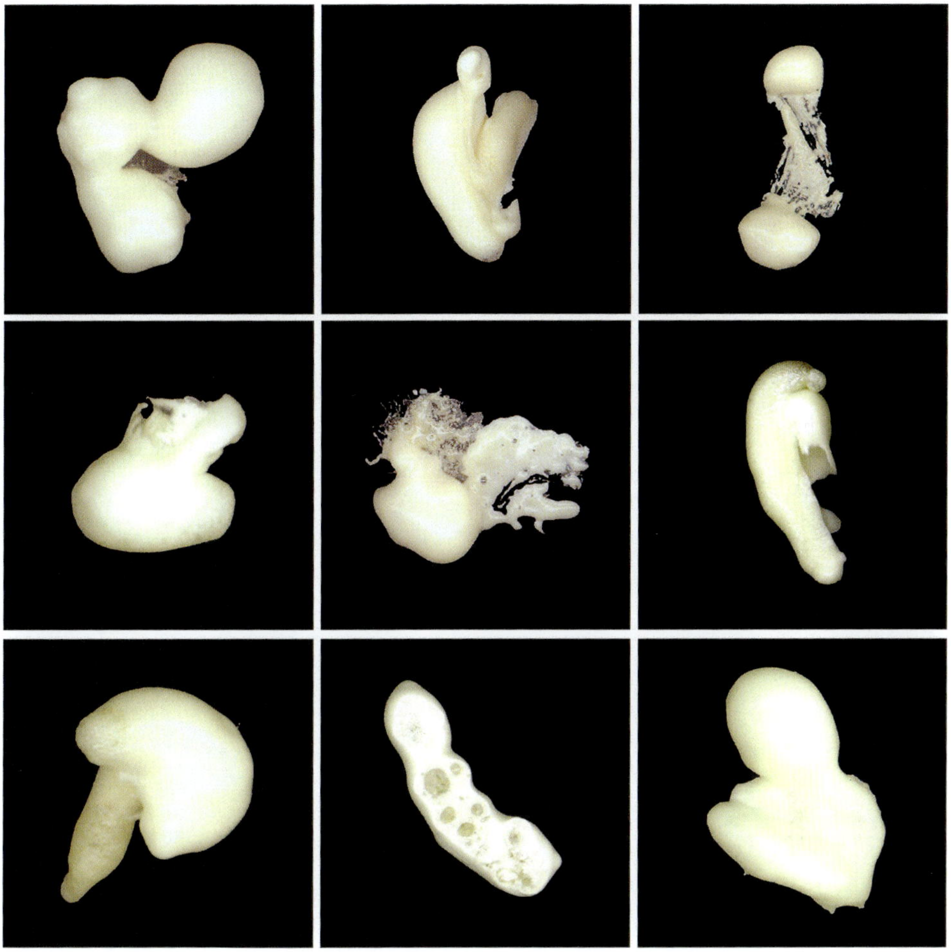

Figure 44. Suzanne Anker, *Stem Cells* series, 2004.
9 archival inkjet prints on paper, 13 x 19 in (33 x 48 cm) each.

Golden Boy, is a slang term referring to a very successful male who has attracted praise and resources at an early age. Although females are attaining positions of power, we still live in a male-dominated society where males have more advantages than females.

SF: Along with your sculptures you also exhibited a number of digital prints. They take the form of body parts and cells. What was your intention here?

SA: The printed images do references stem cells, which have reached celebrity status. These cells have a unique ability to morph into a number of the body's cells such as heart, nerve and even skin cells. Because of their polysemous nature they are regularly employed in scientific research and regenerative medicine.

The *Stem Cells* series (figs. 44,45) evolved as a way to explore how material, whether organic or inorganic, can take a myriad of unique forms. These images began as a series of tiny sculptures constructed from polyurethane foam. Slight differences in applied air pressure acting upon the material delivered various configurations. The forms took on the appearances not only of body parts and cells but also of fetuses and animals. By coaxing materials and processes, even in a slight matter, extreme alterations in shape can occur. Such is the same for stem cells.

References

Anker, Suzanne. 'Cellular Archeology' in "Models, Metaphors, and Matter: Artists and Scientists Visualize Scientific Concepts." *Art Journal* 55, no. 1 (1996): 33-43.

Anker, Suzanne. "Prime Objects and Body Doubles." *Art Journal* 68, no. 4 (1996): 99-104.

Anker, Suzanne, and Dorothy Nelkin. *The Molecular Gaze: Art in the Genetic Age*. Cold Spring Harbor, N.Y.: Cold Spring Harbor Laboratory Press, 2004.

Boxer, Sarah. "At Play With DNA." *The New York Times*, March 14, 2003, 35-39.

Cairns-Smith, A. G. *Seven Clues to the Origin of Life A Scientific Detective Story*. Cambridge [England]: Cambridge University Press, 1990.

Kubler, George Alexander. *The Shape of Time. Remarks on the History of Things*. Yale University Press: New Haven & London, 1962.

Gostin, Lawrence O. *Surrogate Motherhood Politics and Privacy*. Bloomington: Indiana University Press, 1990.

Rorimer, Anne. "Self-Referentiality and Mass-Production in the Work of Allan McCollum, 1969-1989." In *Allan McCollum*. Eindhoven: Stedelijk Van Abbemuseum, 1989.

List of Illustrations

Fig. 38: Suzanne Anker, *Buddha Baby*, from *Origins and Futures*, 2005 (detail). Rapid prototype sculpture of plaster and resin, stainless steel, pyrite minerals, 96 x 96 in (244 x 244 cm). Installation view of *Golden Boy* at Universal Concepts Unlimited, New York City. Photograph by D. James Dee.

Fig. 39: Suzanne Anker, *Origins and Futures*, 2005 (detail). Rapid prototype sculpture of plaster and resin, stainless steel, pyrite minerals, 96 x 96 in (244 x 244 cm). Installation view of *Golden Boy* at Universal Concepts Unlimited, New York City. Photograph by D. James Dee.

Fig. 40: Suzanne Anker, *Origins and Futures*, 2005. Rapid prototype sculpture of plaster and resin, stainless steel, pyrite minerals, 96 x 96 in (244 x 244 cm). Installation view of *FutureNatural* at Deborah Colton Gallery, Houston, Texas.

Fig. 41: Left: Suzanne Anker, *First Fetus*, 2004. Rapid prototype sculpture, urethane foam and acrylic, 25 x 38 x 13 in (63.5 x 96.5 x 33 cm). Right: Suzanne Anker, *Golden Boy*, 2004. Rapid prototype sculpture, urethane foam and acrylic, 16 x 24 x 18 in (40.6 x 61 x 45.7 cm).

Fig. 42: Suzanne Anker, *Cubist Baby*, 2004. Rapid Prototype sculpture, urethane foam and acrylic. 32 x 16 x 16 in (81 x 40 x 40 cm).

Fig. 43: Suzanne Anker, *Stem Cells #4*, 2004. Archival inkjet print on paper, 13 x 19 in (33 x 48 cm).

Fig. 44: Suzanne Anker, *Stem Cells* series, 2004. Nine archival inkjet prints on paper, 13 x 19 in (33 x 48 cm) each.

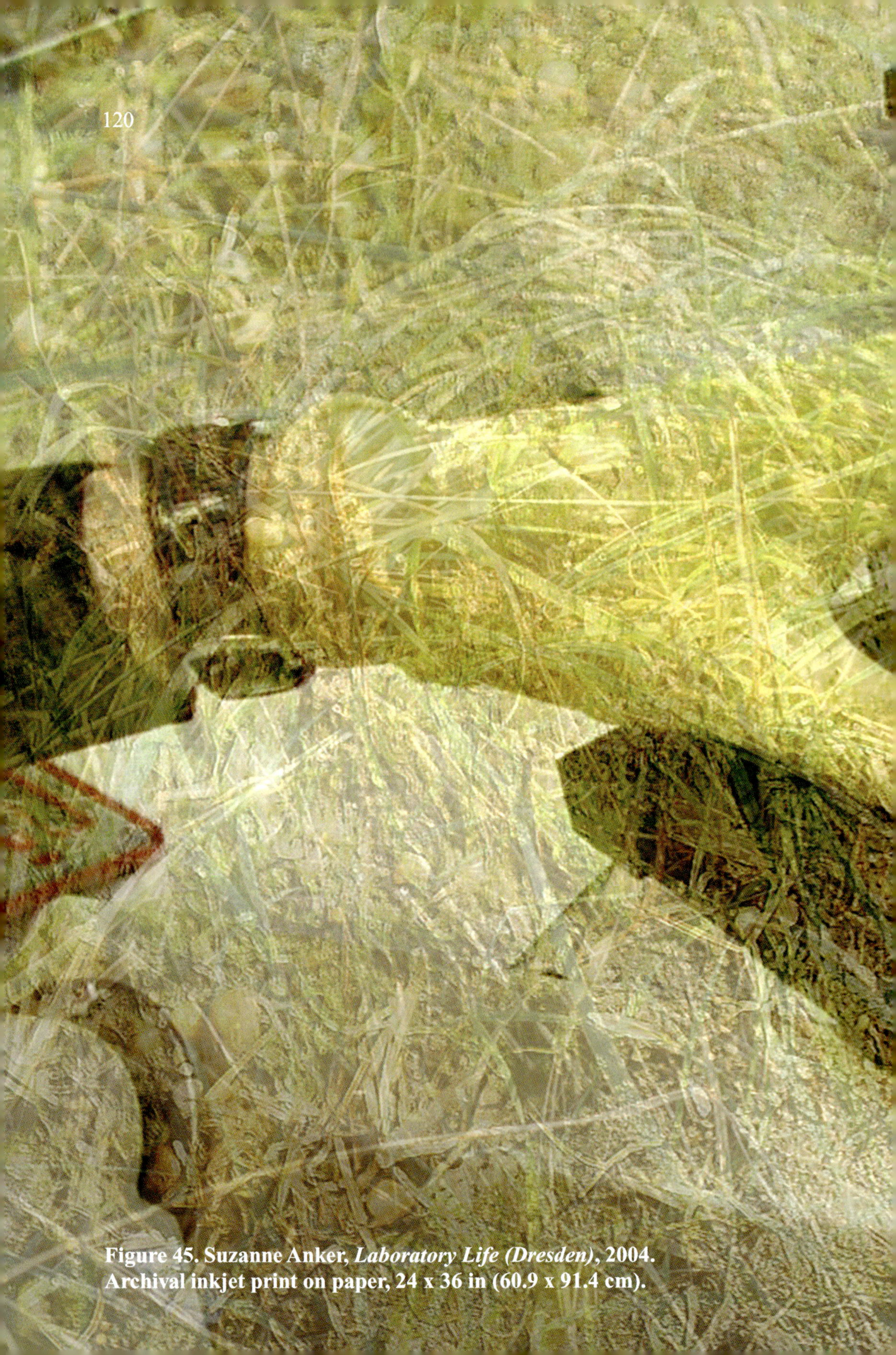

Figure 45. Suzanne Anker, *Laboratory Life (Dresden)*, 2004. Archival inkjet print on paper, 24 x 36 in (60.9 x 91.4 cm).

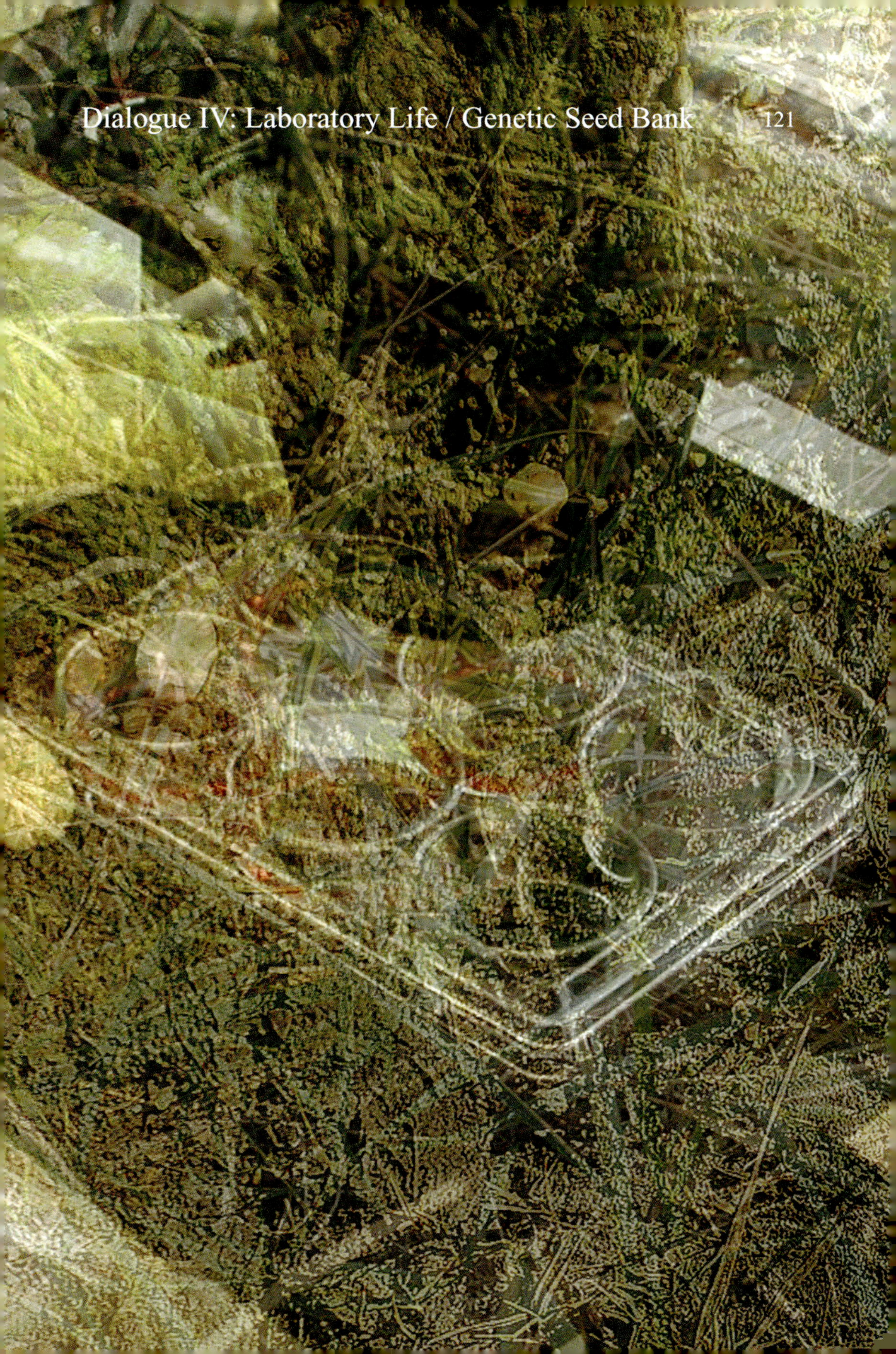

Dialogue IV: Laboratory Life / Genetic Seed Bank

SUZANNE ANKER & SABINE FLACH

Sabine Flach: In *Laboratory Life*, you superimposed images of gardens over photographs of scientific research institutions. Although this technique was executed through Photoshop, it does reference the double exposure as used by the Surrealists in the 1920s and 30s. How does the double exposure function in your work and what part does chance play?

Suzanne Anker: Double exposure as engaged by the Surrealists was an experimental photographic technique intended to produce uncanny images. In effect, it was an unpredictable way of exposing the unconscious, by mechanistic means. Along with photograms and solarization, double exposures expanded photography's graphic capabilities. For example, in Man Ray's portrait *Marquise Casati* (1922), the sitter appears to possess two sets of eyes. While this image is not congruent with reality, psychologically speaking, the portrait is arresting.

In *Laboratory Life* images of gardens and scientific apparatuses mingle, creating a tapestry effect that could not be achieved by a single exposure. In *Laboratory Life (Dresden*) (fig. 45) we see a gloved hand that appears to be made of hay, perhaps a reference to the classic straw man in the *Wizard of Oz*, a character who didn't have a brain. Assuming this is a fortuitous critique of the molecular sciences or just an incidental coincidence, this image could not have been composed by ordinary means. This conceptual mixing and matching produces results that cannot be predicted prior to their overlay. *Laboratory Life (Rome)* (fig. 46) turns ordinary laboratory paraphernalia such as specimen bottles, pipettes and plastic containers into a medley of red, yellow and blue, making reference to the color wheel's primary colors. This compound photograph allowed my thoughts to meander towards Barnett Newman's *Who's Afraid of Red, Yellow and Blue* (1966) and Piet Mondrian's, *Broadway Boogie-Woogie* (1943). Even Damien Hirst has employed this art historical marker to his own ends. In *The Four Elements (Who's Afraid of Red, Yellow, Green and Blue*) (2005), the artist attaches dead butterflies to his four monochromatic paintings. All of these cases point to abstraction's reductive attempts to use primary colors as building blocks in painting and the manner in which images and their ideology are imprinted on memory. The magic in red, yellow and blue, the *ur-colors* of the wheel, are an inherent matrix for producing inordinate numbers of combinatory mixes. They are, in effect, primary building blocks, like molecular gene sequences, for generating vast differences in material applications.

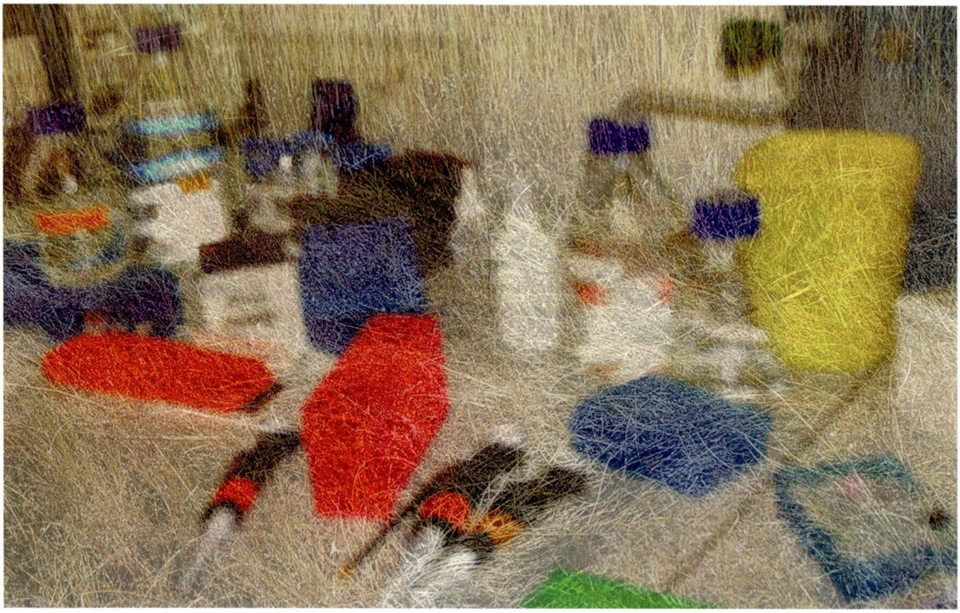

Figure 46. Suzanne Anker, *Laboratory Life (Rome)*, 2006.
Archival inkjet print on paper, 24 x 36 in (60.9 x 91.4 cm).

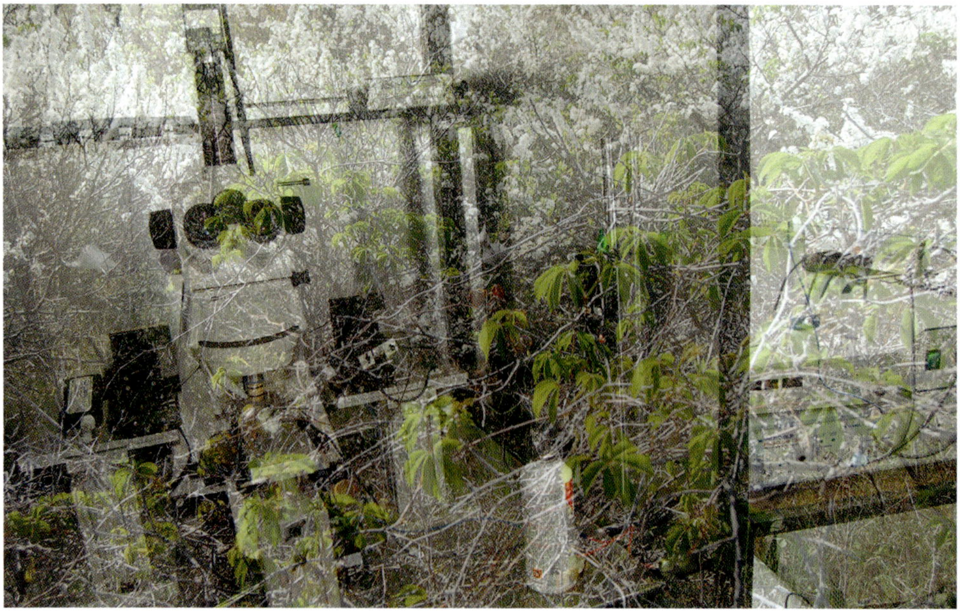

Figure 47. Suzanne Anker, *Laboratory Life (Snowman)*, 2007.
Archival inkjet print on paper, 24 x 36 in (60.9 x 91.4 cm).

SF: What role do laboratories play for you? You have visited and photographed many of them, the European Molecular Biology Laboratory (EMBL) in Rome, the Max Planck Institute in Dresden, a biophysics lab at Imperial College in London. Why is this a recurrent theme in your work? Are laboratories different from artists' studios?

SA: Laboratories are places that have restricted access, like behind-the-scenes specimens in medical collections or private storage rooms in art museums. They are open to the public only by special invitation, ironically making them both collective working spaces and private domains. By photographing each laboratory I was able to compare their differences and similarities, that is, how sub-genres of disciplines such as embryology or biophysics construct their spaces. For example, in *Laboratory Life (Snowman)* (fig. 47) and *Laboratory Life (Biophysics)* (fig. 48) an enormous machine is pictured which measures the electrical charges in a neuron. The image has a dystopic, cyborgian sensibility as a man-made creature takes on a semblance of personhood. The sub-title of this piece, *Snowman,* is a reference to *Oryx and Crake*, Margaret Atwood's speculative realism novel. In *Laboratory Life (Allium)* (fig. 49), plants have infiltrated the lab, canceling out the super potential of precise instrumentation.

Although Big Science's major "appliances" vary, the labeling tools, microscopes, glassware and interior designs are virtually identical. The walls are painted white, the furniture is without ornament, the accoutrements are mostly stainless steel, which include sinks, counters and shelves. This is not true for artists' studios. Artists' spaces have unique sets of working conditions – some are pristine, others retain the indexical marking patterns of former projects, while others merely consist of a desktop computer. Bruno Latour and Steve Woolgar's seminal text *Laboratory Life* provides an account of what actually happens in a laboratory and how scientific facts are created. They also expose the role social interaction plays in scientific discoveries. This exchange does have some resonance with what is termed as a "studio visit," in which curators, critics, gallerists, and other artists participate in an ongoing dialogue. What results from such discussions, in some cases, contributes to the artists' own studio practice. Such "social interaction" functions as a catalyst for developing ideas.

SF: 21st-century laboratories are quite different from laboratories in the past. How would you characterize the differences?

SA: Laboratories in the past housed live animals *in situ*, along with models, charts and instruments. As the sciences developed new disciplines such as molecular and microbiology, the nature and setting of the laboratory changed. Molecular biology, which deals with the cell and its parts, transformed laboratories into more

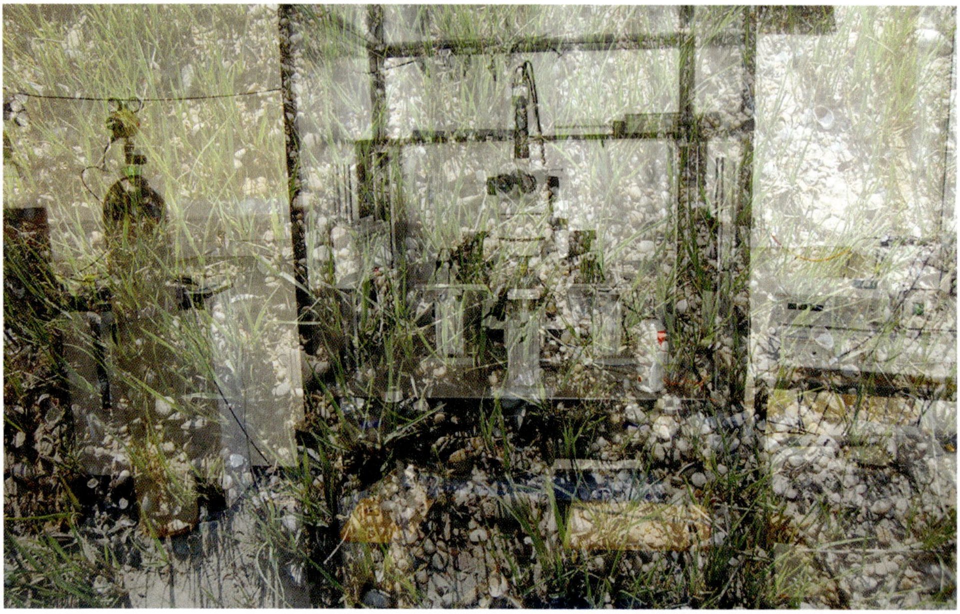

Figure 48. Suzanne Anker, *Laboratory Life (Biophysics)*, 2007.
Archival inkjet print on paper, 24 x 36 in (60.9 x 91.4 cm).

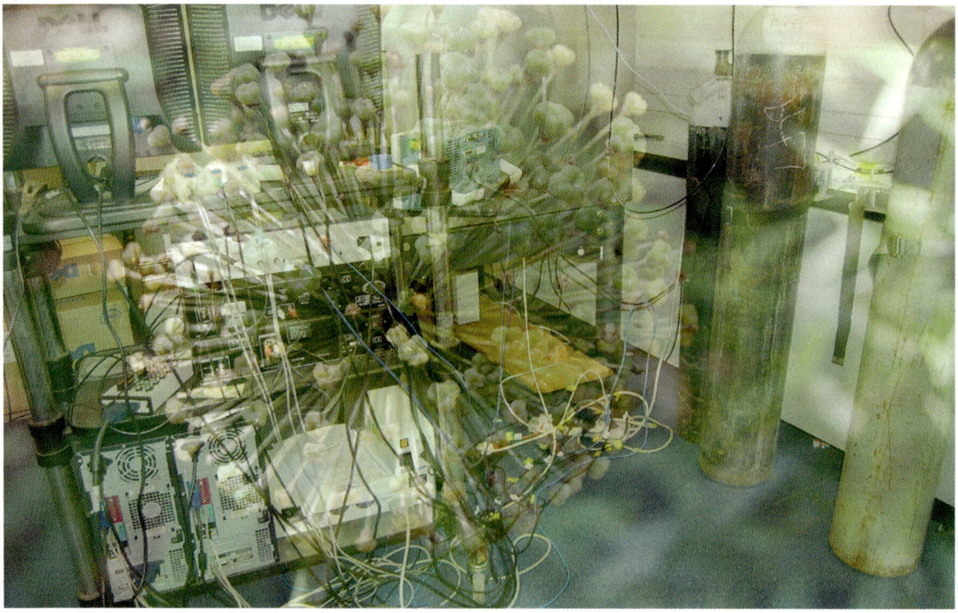

Figure 49. Suzanne Anker, *Laboratory Life (Allium)*, 2007.
Archival inkjet print on paper, 24 x 36 in (60.9 x 91.4 cm).

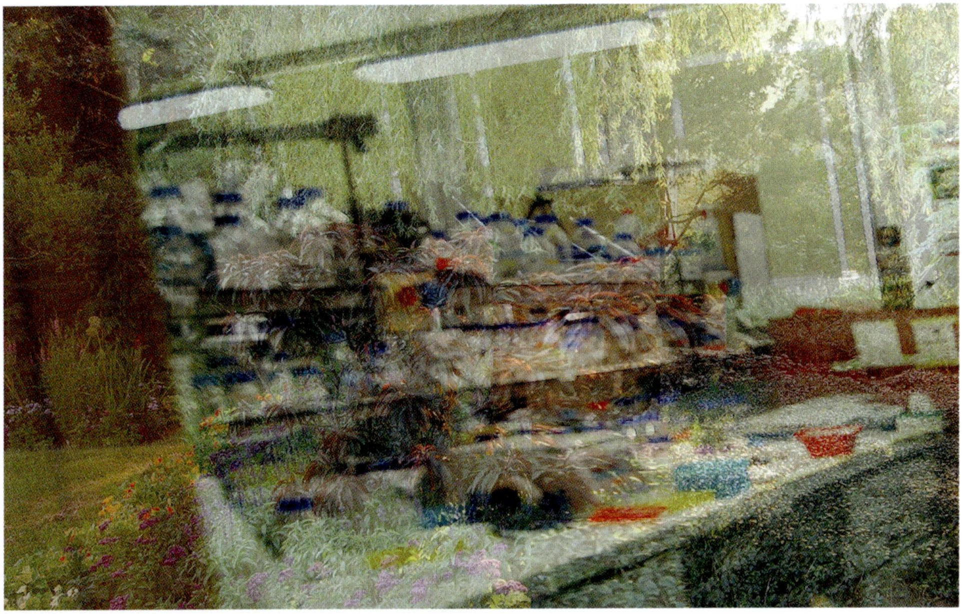

Figure 50. Suzanne Anker, *Laboratory Life (Jump Cut)*, 2006.
Archival inkjet print on paper, 24 x 36 in (60.9 x 91.4 cm).

minimalist "modernized" spaces. Animals are kept separately in places referred to as "animal houses," a derogatory terms attributed to the intense odors arising from these premises. Model organisms such as genetically modified mice, and rats, as well as larger animals such as rabbits are housed in such facilities.

SF: What relationship does a laboratory have to a garden? Does this relationship rest on the ideas of the naturally grown and artificially created?

SA: Both laboratories and gardens are artificially created. They are constructed spaces, framed with either pastoral delight in mind, or as a site where nature is scrutinized, expecting to surrender its secrets, as visualized in *Laboratory Life (Jump Cut)* (fig. 50). Gardens can be playful but also accommodate roving bands of plant and animal life: seeds, insects, birds, moles, and even turtles. There is no possible containment for a garden. Fences cannot keep airborne substances out of its sanctioned space. Gardens function as a slice of arcadia where nature on the surface seems to be cultivated. Laboratories require stricter controls so as not to contaminate research results and are equipped with sealed doors, sterilization units and filtered air.

These open and closed practices, being in the nature/culture nexus, represent current osmotic flow as each side inches towards the other's domain. As nature becomes "culturized," that is, manipulated and transformed, culture absorbs and expands upon these changes. Foodstuffs, pharmaceuticals, and synthetic chemicals are a few of the products of this exchange.

What gardens do in fact have in common with laboratories is the everyday care needed to sustain life. Nature is in continual flux, repositioning its elements constantly. In both gardens and laboratories, caretakers of various sorts are required to maintain proper conditions for each.

SF: You mentioned the piece *Laboratory Life (Jump Cut)*. Originally employed by Jean-Luc Godard in his film *Breathless* (original title: *À bout de souffle*) the jump cut interrupts narrative illusion and creates a reflexive moment. The idyllic images of gardens – with a bounty of forests and flowers – creates a discontinuity in time as digital pixels weave into new threads. How is this notion reflected in your work?

SA: Photography at this point in time has no discrete boundaries. From documentary stills to studio setups, to process-based iconography and its abstract components, from cell phone photography to large format pictures, all genres and techniques are open. Photography's mandate as a slice of reality has also been forfeited. It is another plastic medium like painting or drawing and can be revisioned to suit expectation and aesthetic judgment. Photography is a mechanism of recording, much like sketchbooks were during the last century.

The "jump cut" is so pervasive in our lives that we rarely notice it. Just pick up a newspaper or watch a TV program, bookended by commercials. We go from news coverage about the war in Iraq to the most up-to-the-minute facial cream, without blinking an eye. These point and shoot applications can be bracketed, layered, or even repetitive, as content is moved instantaneously from one position to another in real time.

SF: Do you see your studio as a kind of laboratory in which different components, objects, impressions and ideas flow together?

SA: Yes, of course. Everything in my studio functions as source material for my work: books, music, media, models, paints, plaster, tools, cloth, glassware, plants, tables, light sources, cameras, prints, computers and other thinking devices. It is a location that serves as a spatial template for installations, past and future. How ideas germinate cannot be predetermined. One can only speculate on the ways in which artworks come to fruition.

SF: Let's turn our attention to another laboratory, this time one specializing in researching and reclaiming coral. When you visited the Mote Tropical Research Laboratory in the Florida Keys, you were introduced to specimens of coral in

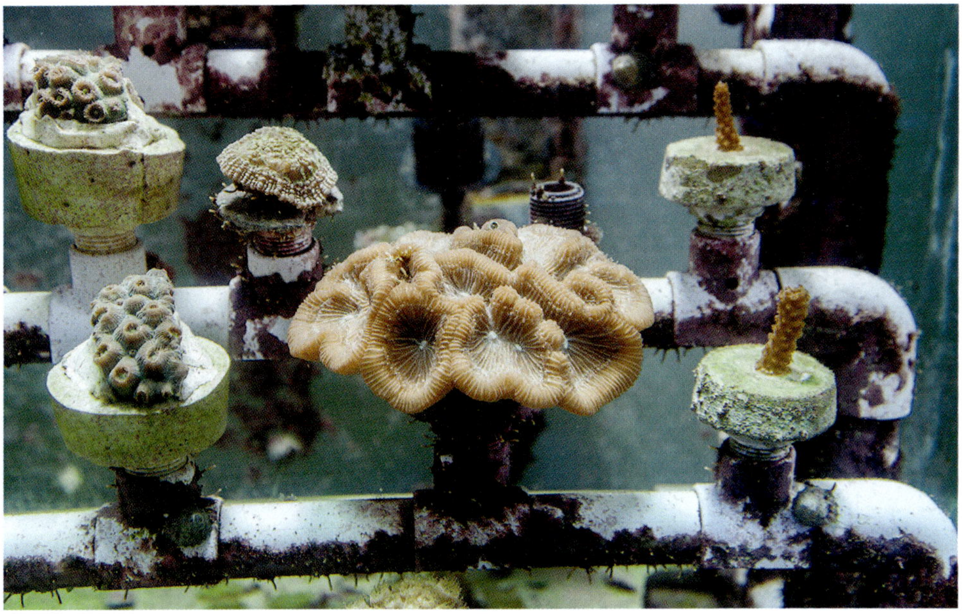

Figure 51. Suzanne Anker, *Genetic Seed Bank (Big Brain)*, 2007.
Archival inkjet print on paper, 24 x 36 in (60.9 x 91.4 cm).

glass tanks. This visit provided the source material for *Genetic Seed Bank.* Please talk about that series of work.

SA: Genetic information is a decisive tool for investigating life forms and their relationships. Many genomes of both animals and plants have not yet been deciphered and coral is one of those species. Coral exists in many varieties, some of which are carnivorous and others that create symbiotic relationships with plants. In the latter case, sunlight is a catalytic mechanism for the chlorophyll in plants to undergo photosynthesis. This process creates food for the distinct, yet intertwined, polyps. During the 19th century, coral was erroneously considered a plant, but that classification has since been corrected.

SF: The tanks housing the coral are quite unique in design. They are not the kind of artifacts readily seen in aquariums. What is their purpose at this institute?

SA: After considerable trial and error, the decision to use PVC pipes as a substructure to house the coral specimens in unique tanks seemed most appropriate. The plastic piping is inexpensive and suitable for water submersion since it normally functions as plumbing pipes. Here the pipes are designed as a matrix onto which small concrete "pedestals" hold the corals in place, as is shown in *Genetic*

Seed Bank (Big Brain) (fig. 51), *Genetic Seed Bank (Palmata)* (fig. 52), *Genetic Seed Bank (Purple-Algae)* (fig. 53) and *Genetic Seed Bank (White Cloud)* (figs. 54-55). This framework allows researchers to accurately record the growth patterns and health of each specimen. Each fragment of coral is furnished with an ongoing, recorded history, that is, where they were found, the conditions of their in-situ environment, and to what species they belong.

SF: Please discuss your invocation of a seed bank in this work.

SA: These specimens do in fact function as seeds. They have been acquired by the lab for study and analysis. When they reach a certain size and other determinations have been made, they are relocated back into the ocean hoping they can continue to regenerate. Each coral is firmly placed on small concrete slabs on the ocean floor.

SF: Coral appeared as an important species in both Darwin's work and early *Wunderkammer*. What is the attraction to this entity?

SA: These images represent what can be referred to as a living *Wunderkammer*. Whereas the coral presented in historical *Wunderkammer* are dead and dried fragments, these specimens retain their life functions. Submerged in life-supporting aquarium tanks, they continue their existence as creatures of study under enhanced conditions. For Darwin, coral reefs were instrumental in leading him to his controversial theory of evolution. *The Structure and Distribution of Coral Reefs* (1842), was the first monograph he published, which recorded his research from his voyage on the *Beagle*.

SF: What function does coral play in global ecosystems?

SA: Coral reefs are complete ecosystems consisting of fish and plants in addition to the coral itself. They are communities of organisms interacting with one another. When a coral reef is destroyed by temperature changes or pollution, the entire constellation of living forms is affected. Corals themselves are composed of polyps, which work together to form an organism. Like heart cells that beat in unison, they are small entities that make up an organ-like structure.

SF: From an aesthetic point of view, how do you see these images in relation to your other work?

SA: As specimens under glass, this work extends my investigation into glass-enclosed once-living forms. As fragmented body parts, they are, in effect, historical entities pointing to the scientific and cultural aspects of a given time.

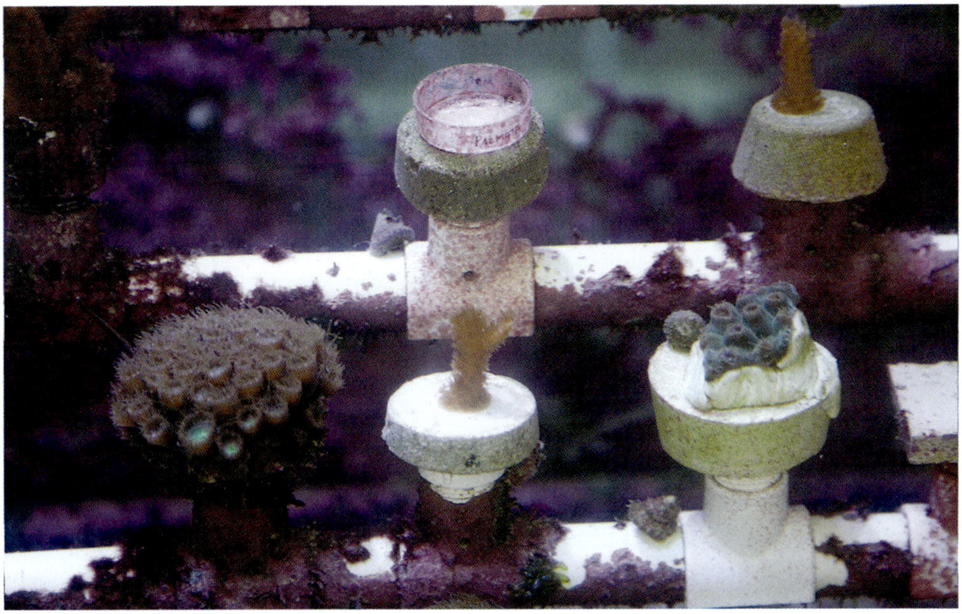

Figure 52. Suzanne Anker, *Genetic Seed Bank (Palmata)*, 2007.
Archival inkjet print on paper, 24 x 36 in (60.9 x 91.4 cm).

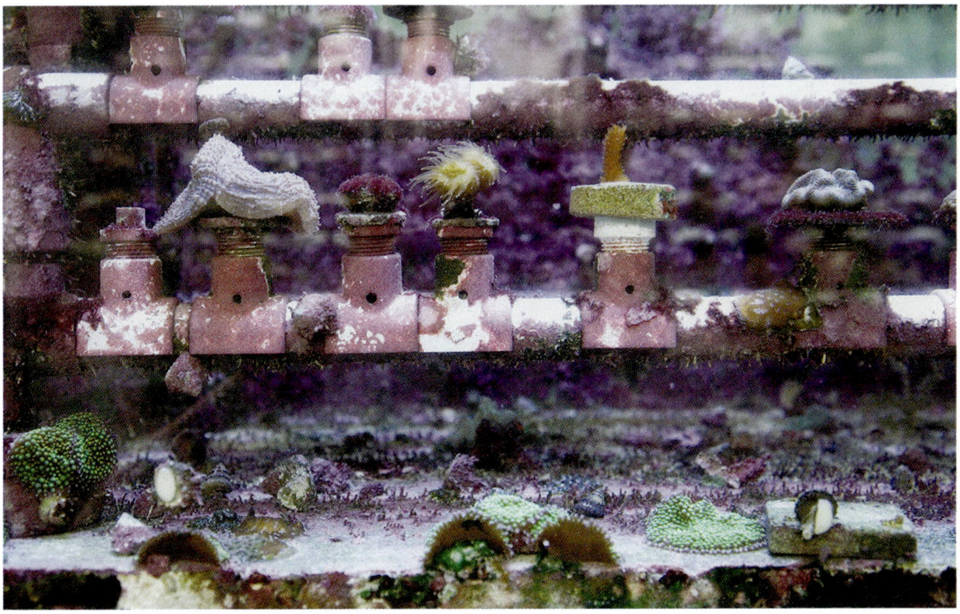

Figure 53. Suzanne Anker, *Genetic Seed Bank (Purple-Algae)*, 2007.
Archival inkjet print on paper, 24 x 36 in (60.9 x 91.4 cm).

I have also created an animation from one of my still photographs from this series. The work is presented as a large-scale video projection in a darkened room. The one-minute animation is on a loop, and moves extremely slowly, almost imperceptibly, but not quite so (figs. 56, 57). The viewer is brought into a hallucinatory world where his perception is challenged by the mutable aspects of the image itself. The tank appears to be moving as it does rightfully so in an aquarium, however, the scale of the tank under these viewing conditions simultaneously creates an underwater experience.

References

Atwood, Margaret. *Oryx and Crake: A Novel.* New York: Nan A. Talese, 2003.

Breathless / À bout de souffle (original title). Directed by Jean-Luc Godard. 1960. Rialto Pictures, Film.

Colour, edited by David Batchelor. London: Whitechapel; MIT: Boston, 2008.

Darwin, Charles. *The Structure and Distribution of Coral Reefs.* Berkeley: University of California Press, 1962.

Finlay, Victoria. *Color: A Natural History of the Palette.* New York: Random House, 2003.

Latour, Bruno, and Steve Woolgar. *Laboratory Life: The Construction of Scientific Facts.* Princeton, N.J.: Princeton University Press, 1986.

List of Illustrations

Fig. 45: Suzanne Anker, *Laboratory Life (Dresden)*, 2004. Archival inkjet print on paper, 24 x 36 in (60.9 x 91.4 cm).

Fig. 46: Suzanne Anker, *Laboratory Life (Rome)*, 2006. Archival inkjet print on paper, 24 x 36 in (60.9 x 91.4 cm).

Fig. 47: Suzanne Anker, *Laboratory Life (Snowman)*, 2007. Archival inkjet print on paper, 24 x 36 in (60.9 x 91.4 cm).

Fig. 48: Suzanne Anker, *Laboratory Life (Biophysics)*, 2007. Archival inkjet print on paper, 24 x 36 in (60.9 x 91.4 cm).

Fig. 49: Suzanne Anker, *Laboratory Life (Allium)*, 2007. Archival inkjet print on paper, 24 x 36 in (60.9 x 91.4 cm).

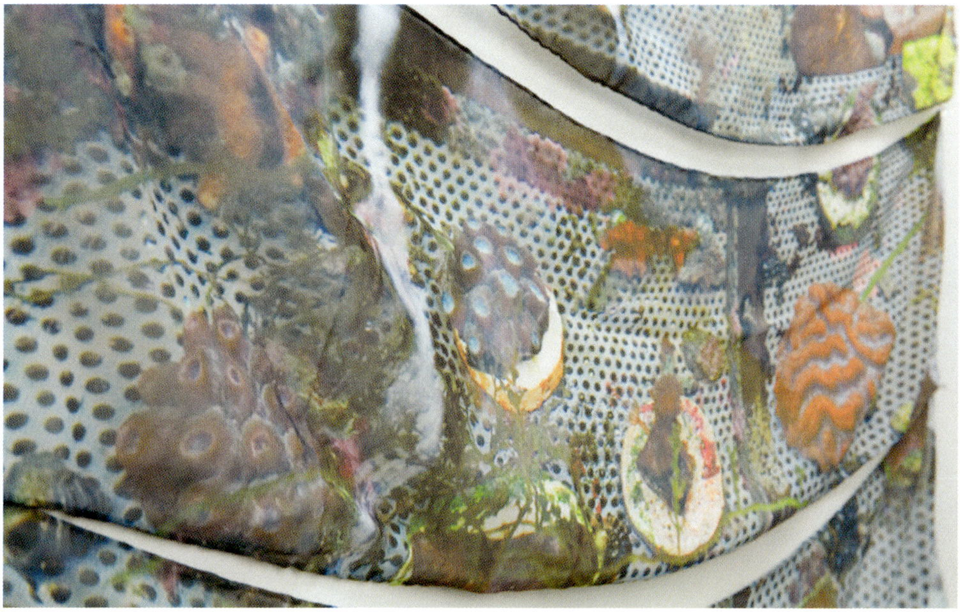

Figure 54. Suzanne Anker, *Genetic Seed Bank (White Cloud)*, 2014. Inkjet print on translucent fabric, hand-sewn stitched border. Three panels of 12.5 x 54 in (31.75 x 137.2 cm) each.

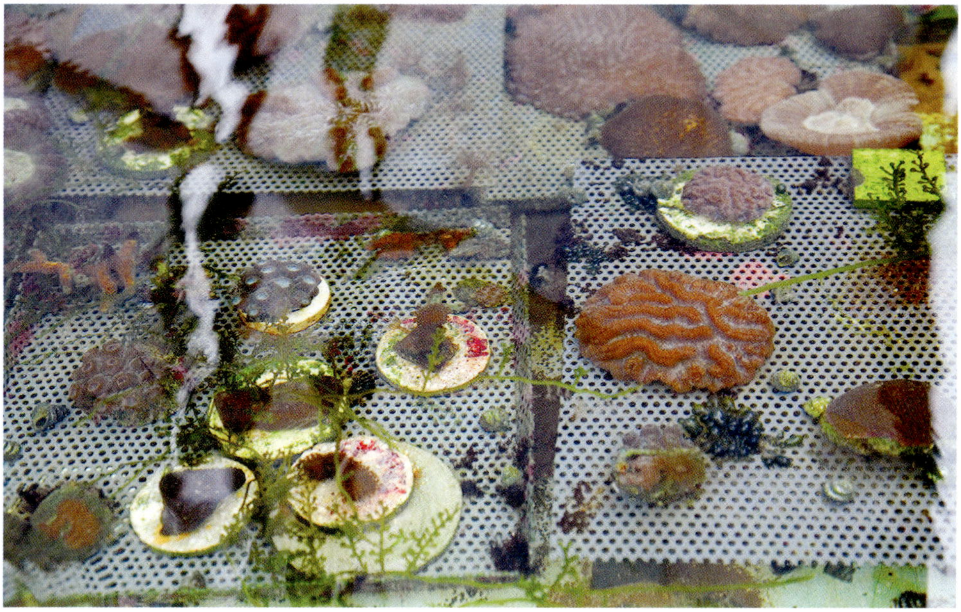

Figure 55. Suzanne Anker, *Genetic Seed Bank (White Cloud)*, 2007.
Archival inkjet print on paper, 24 x 36 in (60.9 x 91.4 cm).

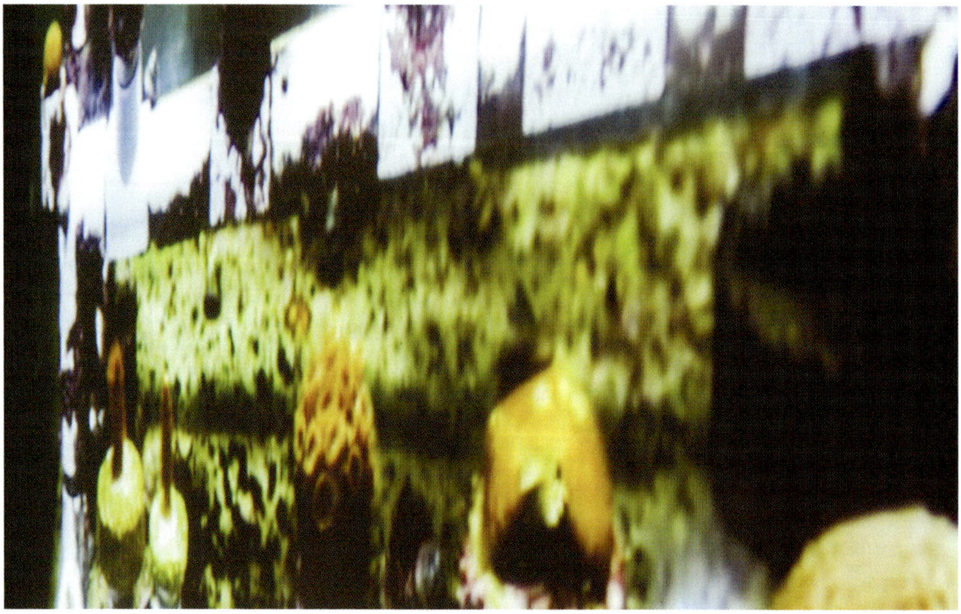

Figure 56. Suzanne Anker, installation view of *Genetic Seed Bank*, 2007 (detail). Single-channel video (color, silent), 1 min looped. Photograph by Raul Valverde.

Fig. 50: Suzanne Anker, *Laboratory Life (Jump Cut)*, 2006. Archival inkjet print on paper, 24 x 36 in (60.9 x 91.4 cm).

Fig. 51: Suzanne Anker, *Genetic Seed Bank (Big Brain)*, 2007. Archival inkjet print on paper, 24 x 36 in (60.9 x 91.4 cm).

Fig. 52: Suzanne Anker, *Genetic Seed Bank (Palmata)*, 2007. Archival inkjet print on paper, 24 x 36 in (60.9 x 91.4 cm).

Fig. 53: Suzanne Anker, *Genetic Seed Bank (Purple-Algae)*, 2007. Archival inkjet print on paper, 24 x 36 in (60.9 x 91.4 cm).

Fig. 54: Suzanne Anker, *Genetic Seed Bank (White Cloud)*, 2014. Inkjet print on translucent fabric, hand-sewn stitched border. Three panels of 12.5 x 54 in (31.75 x 137.2 cm) each.

Fig. 55: Suzanne Anker, *Genetic Seed Bank (White Cloud)*, 2007. Archival inkjet print on paper, 24 x 36 in (60.9 x 91.4 cm).

Fig. 56: Suzanne Anker, installation view of *Genetic Seed Bank*, 2007. (detail) Single-channel video (color, silent), 1 min looped. Photograph by Raul Valverde.

Fig. 57: Suzanne Anker, installation view of *Genetic Seed Bank*, 2007. Single-channel video (color, silent), 1 min looped. Photograph by Raul Valverde.

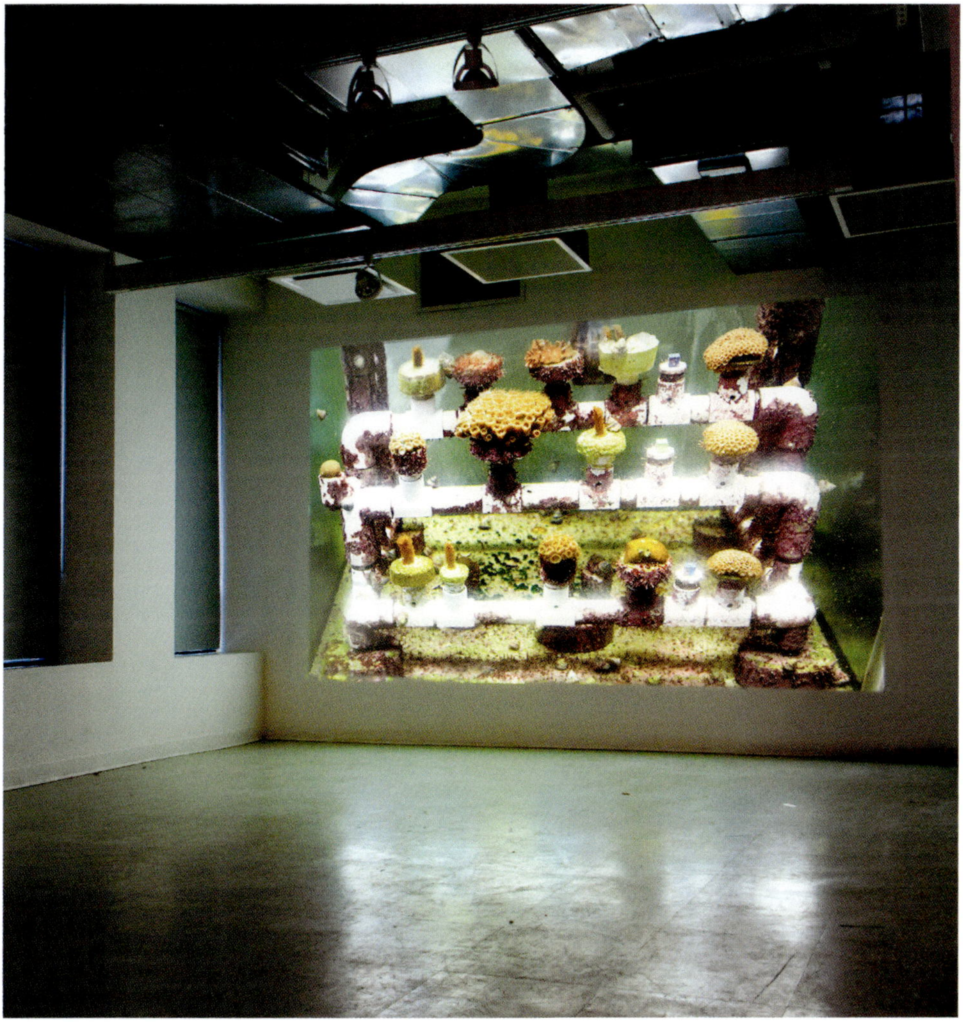

Figure 57. Suzanne Anker, installation view of *Genetic Seed Bank*, 2007. Single-channel video (color, silent), 1 min looped. Photograph by Raul Valverde.

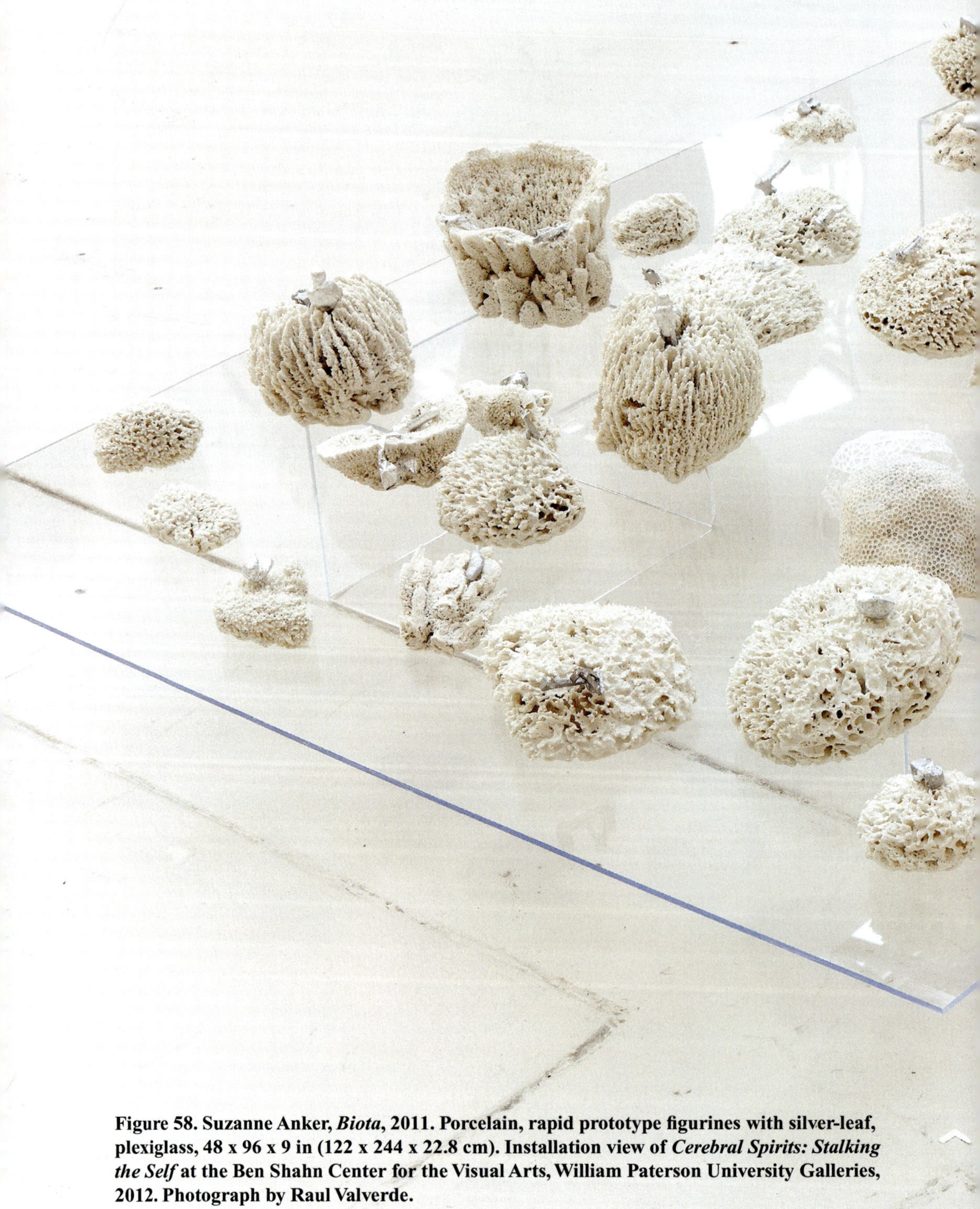

Figure 58. Suzanne Anker, *Biota*, 2011. Porcelain, rapid prototype figurines with silver-leaf, plexiglass, 48 x 96 x 9 in (122 x 244 x 22.8 cm). Installation view of *Cerebral Spirits: Stalking the Self* at the Ben Shahn Center for the Visual Arts, William Paterson University Galleries, 2012. Photograph by Raul Valverde.

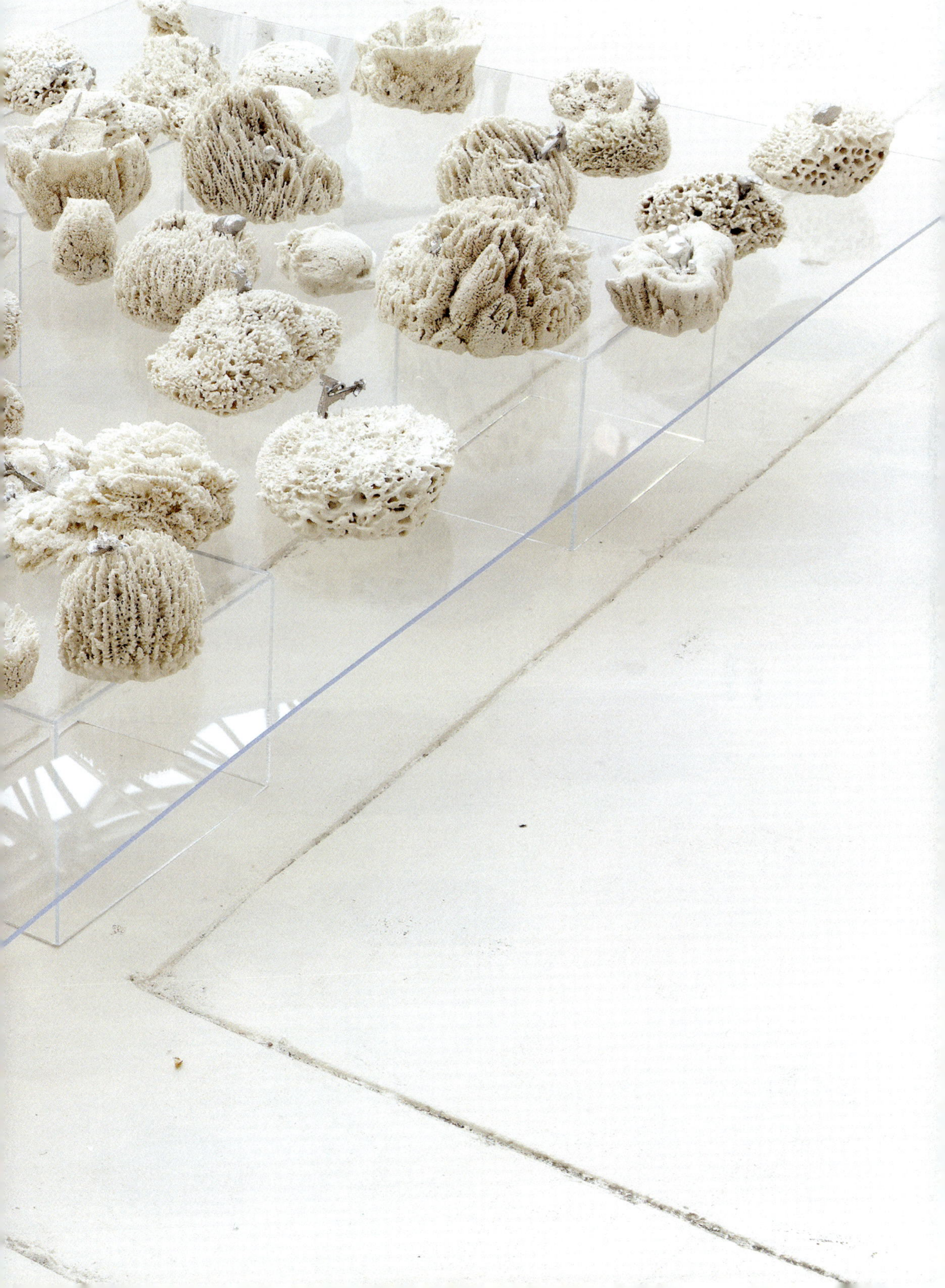

Dialogue V: Biota / Carbon Collision of the Diamond Mind

SUZANNE ANKER & SABINE FLACH

Sabine Flach: *Biota* is an expansive series of porcelain sculptures which you arrange in an installation format. How do you see your sculpture in relation to your other work?

Suzanne Anker: I am primarily a sculptor, a maker of objects. I think in three-dimensions. Perhaps it is the haptic nature of my work, which is replete with textural surfaces, allowing me to relate my sculpture to a corporeal self. Touching and molding material is an alchemical process, as materials go through a measure of becoming something other. Recently, my preoccupation with rapid prototype sculpture simultaneously grants me multiple views of my work from a frontal perspective. Such leverage adds to the ways that dimensionality of matter can be conceptualized. Matter as substance speaks to a consummate kinesthetic experience, in contrast to painting or photography. It is more tangible, more real, closer to the earth-bound elements of gravity and space and how they are displaced.

In two-dimensional work, illusion carries perceptual weight, while in sculpture, there is less presumed ambiguity. We know that sculpture is a thing in space; it is physical, yet metaphorical. It is this dissonance between matter and its incorporated associative meanings, its internal languages, that permits sculpture to enter consciousness as a contradiction. When we encounter matter, we perceive it as a bundle of molecules holding its place in space. We distinguish it as mass. We also become aware of the fact that sculpture is not only composed of matter, but it is a specialized object, akin, but different from an artifact.

SF: Our visit at the last dOCUMENTA (13) in 2012 included work that employed animals. As an art historian it is noteworthy to remark that the status of the animal in art has changed from the late 60s and early 70s. The animal has become integrated into the artwork itself. Where do you see yourself in this development?
SA: Are you talking about Pierre Huyghe's untitled piece which included a dog whose leg was painted bright pink? How is this different from Joseph Beuy's *I Like America and America Likes Me* (1974)–his installation with a coyote? Many artists have included live animals in their works. Matthew Barney's exhibition *The Cremaster Cycle* at the Guggenheim Museum in New York City in 2003 included a live bird. However, the avian was not well cared for and laid prostrate on the gallery's floor near the exit door. Sentient creatures have been employed as accessories to elaborate installation formats. Most recently, Chinese artist Cai

Guo-Qiang's installation *Moving Ghost Town* (2014) at the Aspen Art Museum in Colorado created much controversy about the treatment of animals in artworks. The artist mounted iPads onto the backs of African Sulcata tortoises, which displayed a video of surrounding ghost towns. Many artists have employed dead animals as well in their installations, either in formaldehyde or as taxidermied specimens. From Robert Rauschenberg to Damien Hirst to Maurizio Cattelan, dead animals appear as *objets d'art.* Can we consider Gunter von Hagens' plastinated bodies in this context? My works *Biota* (figs. 58, 59) and *Collision of the Diamond Mind* (figs. 60-62) employ sea and tube sponges as raw matrices which are converted into porcelain. Each sponge is already dead before it is transformed into its ceramic spirit.

SF: Could you describe your interest in animals such as sea sponges and corals?

SA: I am attracted to these creatures because of their detailed beauty and intricate structures. The sea sponge's multicellular animal configuration and the coral's ability to live in communities are intriguing attributes that allow them to work in harmony with their constituent parts, whether they are cells or polyps.

SF: What brought you to the decision to use sponges in particular?

SA: I am very particular with regard to what I consider to be "redeemable metaphors." They are metaphors that have not been exhausted and are multi-coded. In representing the brain and its attendant nervous system as symbolic sources of neuroscientific allegories, metaphors are aesthetically limited. Trees, of course, have been employed by numbers of artists stemming from the exquisite drawings of Santiago Ramón y Cajal, one of the fathers of neuroscience. British artist Andrew Carnie and American sculptor Rona Pondick have successfully employed such imagery as symbols in their work. Branching trees and roots appear in similar configurations as axons and dendrites, the brain's neuronal hardwire responsible for synapses. However, I identified the sea sponge as a perfect metaphor for the brain, since they filter what passes through them. They soak up what comes their way, like a human brain does, as it senses material worlds.

Sponges, like brains, are all individual and unique, varying in kind and complexity. They are ancient forms of life, arising hundreds of millions of years ago as one of the first multicellular animals. Recently, research has shown the significance of the sea sponge's genome. It is a model creature for understanding the necessary cooperation between cells working together in order to create a complicated organism. If unison is not accomplished, the physical results are disastrous. For scientists such as Daniel Rokhsar, a professor of genetics, genomics and development at the University of California, Berkeley, "multicellularity and cancer are two sides of the same coin." In deciphering the sponge's genome, it was found that a multiplicity of genes which cause cancer in humans are also present in sea sponges.[1] Since sea sponges have created mechanisms whereby cells do not overproliferate, but act as a coordinated whole, they hold clues to understanding malignant cell growth in cancer.

Research into anti-cancer drugs is also being conducted by Dr. Matthew Fuchter and his team at Imperial College London, an institution I visited on one of my excursions where I produced *Laboratory Life.* A naturally occurring substance called psammaplin A, present in the sea sponge, is a chemical which extinguishes the rogue growth of cancer cells.[2] As a form of synthetic biology, scientists are adjusting this chemical compound to create structural variations. Thus, its isolation as a naturally occurring compound has spawned artificial varieties of this chemical to combat out-of-control cell growth.

Other novel pharmaceuticals are being developed by mimicking the sea sponge's response to predators. As a – mostly – stationary creature, unable to bite or run, the sea sponge protects itself by forming symbiotic relationships with bacteria and fungi.[3] By studying the compounds produced by this interspecies relationship, researchers at Tel Aviv University under the direction of Micha Ilan are working on the creation of new forms of anti-resistant antibiotics.

Although these ancient multicellar animals lack nervous systems, marine sponges offer clues to the developmental origins of complex neurological systems. Sea sponges possess "signature proteins" which react like those functioning in synapses although they have no neurons. They possess all of the building blocks for the development of nerves, which make them invaluable organisms for studying neurological disorders such as Parkinson's, Alzheimer's and Amyotrophic lateral sclerosis[4]. Although, of course, we don't look or act like sea sponges,

1 Robert Sanders, "Genome of Ancient Sponge Reveals Origins of First Animals, Cancer," *UC Berkeley NewsCenter: News from the University of California, Berkeley* (blog). August 4, 2010.

2 Tel Aviv University, "Common Marine Sponges May Provide Super-antibiotics Of The Future," *ScienceDaily*, March 4, 2009.

3 Ibid.

4 See MA Bruno, F. Pellas, and S. Laureys, "Quality of Life in Locked-in Syndrome Survivors," In *Yearbook of Intensive Care and Emergency Medicine 2008*, ed. J. L Vincent, 881-890. (Berlin: Springer, 2008). Pseudocoma or locked-in syndrome was first described by Plum and Posner in 1966. The patient with locked-in syndrome is fully conscious but interaction with the external world is very limited. Usually, but not always, the anatomy of the responsible lesion in the brainstem is such that locked-in syndrome patients are left with the capacity to use vertical eye movements and blinking to communicate. The earliest example of a 'locked-in patient' was described in 1854 in Alexandre Dumas' novel *The Count of Monte Cristo*. Some years later, Zola described a woman who was paralyzed and "buried alive in a dead body" but could communicate via eye movements in his book *Thérèse Raquin*. Dumas and Zola thus described the locked-in syndrome before the medical community did.

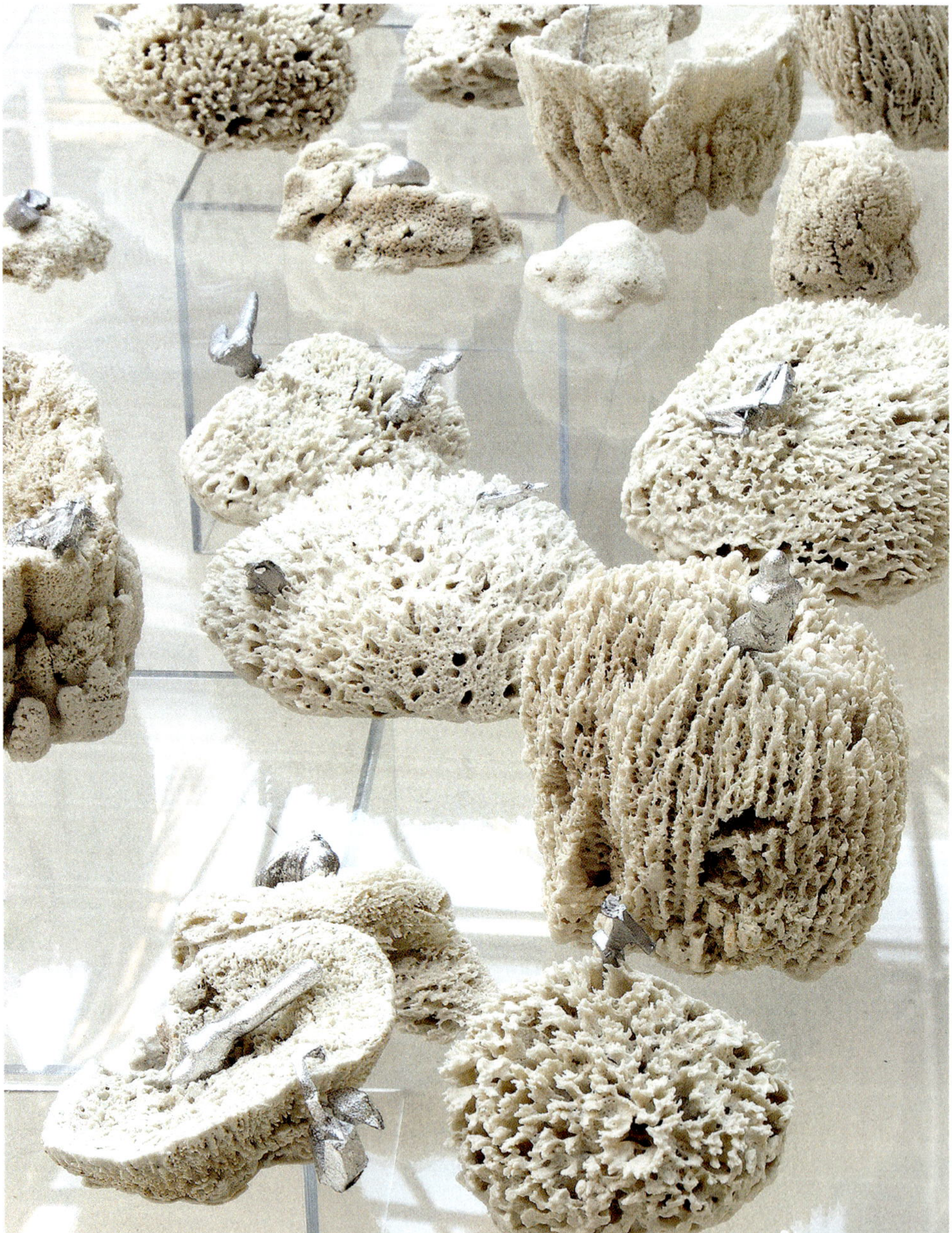

Figure 59. Suzanne Anker, *Biota*, 2011 (detail). Porcelain, rapid prototype figurines with silver-leaf, plexiglass, 48 x 96 x 9 in (122 x 244 x 22.8 cm). Installation view of *Cerebral Spirits: Stalking the Self* at the Ben Shahn Center for the Visual Arts, William Paterson University Galleries, 2012. Photograph by Raul Valverde.

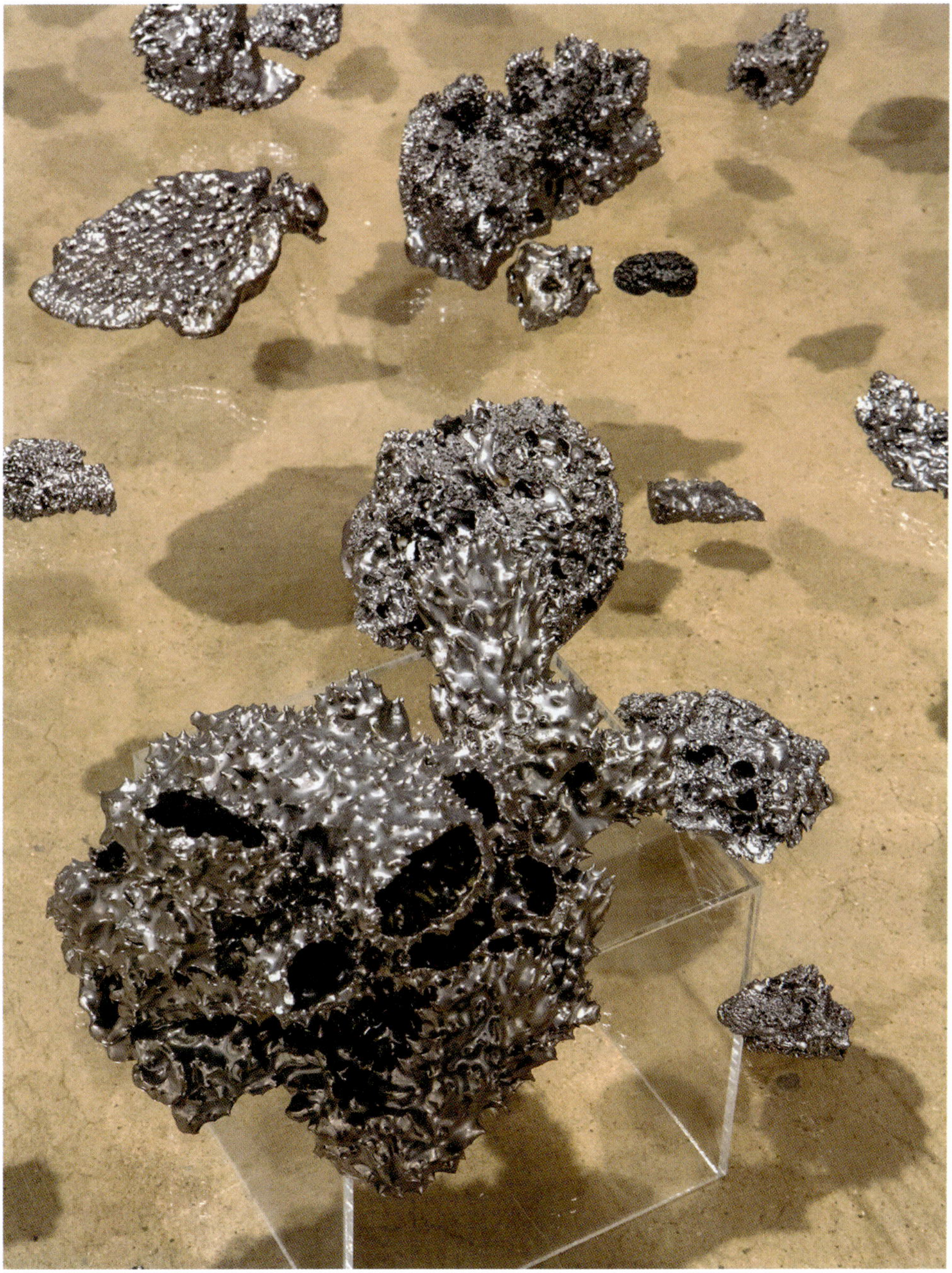

Figure 60. Suzanne Anker, *Carbon Collision In the Diamond Mind*, 2013 (detail). Metallic-glazed porcelain, plexiglass, 48 x 96 x 9 in (122 x 244 x 22.8 cm). Installation view of *While Darkness Sleeps* at the McKinney Avenue Contemporary (The MAC), Dallas, Texas. Photograph by Fernando Rojas.

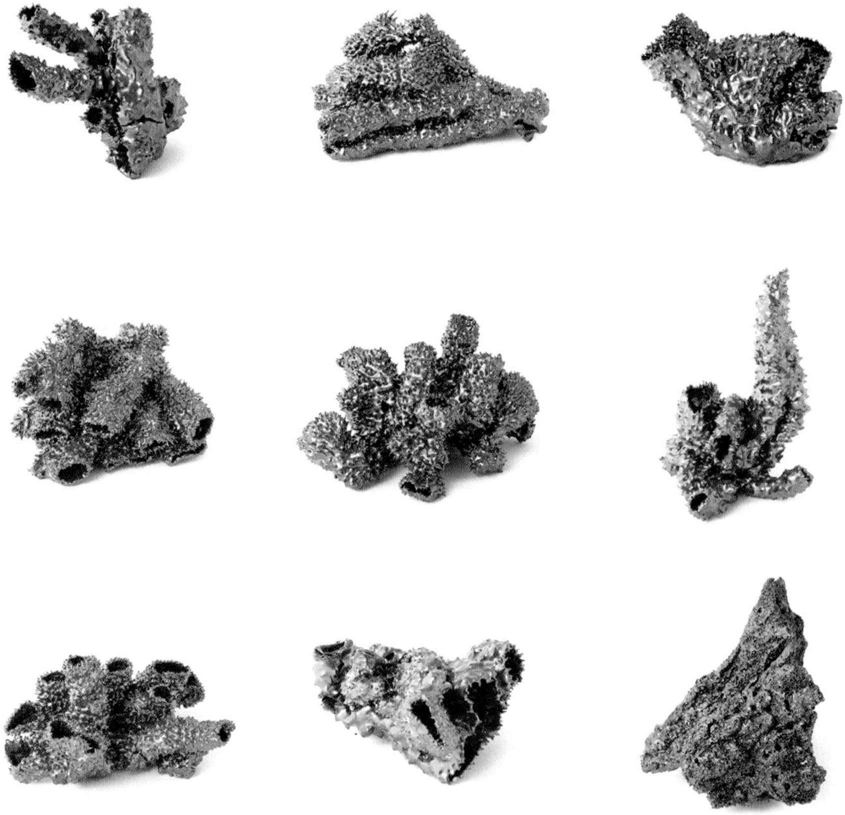

Figure 61. Suzanne Anker, Metallic-glazed porcelain sculptures from the *Carbon Collision In the Diamond Mind* installation, 2013. Photographs by Raul Valverde.

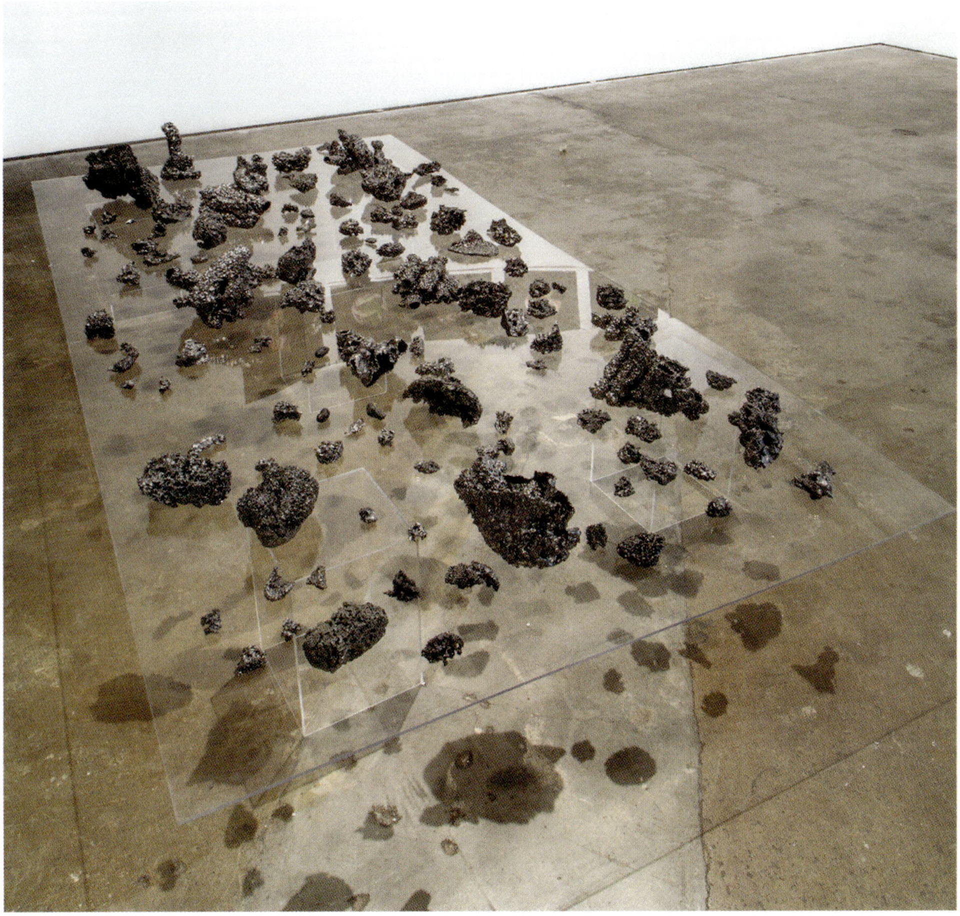

Figure 62. Suzanne Anker. *Carbon Collision In the Diamond Mind*, 2013 (detail). Metallic-glazed porcelain, plexiglass, 48 x 96 x 9 in (122 x 244 x 22.8 cm). Installation view of *FotoFest: Remote Sensing: Microlandscapes and Untold Stories* at Deborah Colton Gallery, Houston, Texas, 2014. Photograph by Henry G. Sanchez.

as humans we share seventy percent of their genes. Even the venerable American poet, Emily Dickinson, has remarked on the sponge's congruity to the brain:

> The brain is wider than the sky,
> For put them side by side,
> The one the other will include
> With ease, and you beside.
>
> The brain is deeper than the sea
> For, hold them, blue to blue,
> The one the other will absorb,
> As sponges, buckets, do
>
> The brain is just the weight of God,
> For lift them, pound for pound,
> And they will differ, if they do,
> As syllable from sound.

SF: Could you please explain why you inserted little silver figurines into the porcelain sponges?

SA: Figurative sculpture is attributed by various theories to neuronal changes in the brains of early humans approximately 200,000 years ago. As a form of mimesis and ritual, such a figurative turn may have also been the result of a change in consciousness (figs. 63-65). The figures represented here are modeled after early "Venus" statuettes and were evidence to anthropologists, paleontologists and archaeologists of an already rich flourishing culture, which included art and musical instruments, more than 35,000 years ago. More recently, the discovery of a "Venus" figure was found "below three feet of sediment in the Hohle Fels Cave, in Germany" (fig. 66). This new find is reported to be the oldest figurative statue yet discovered. For archaeologists it represents evolutionary clues concerning the period in which there was an intermingling of Neanderthals and modern humans. In addition we can think about the Neanderthals as our "kissing cousins" since current DNA analysis can record common percentages of Neanderthal ancestry in a person's genome.

Alternately, it has been speculated that there exists a correspondence between animal brains–trout, frogs, alligators, rabbits et al. and the demarcations of form in ancient figurines.[5] This is something I noticed in 2010 when I gazed at an acrylic

5 Bethe Hagens, "Venuses, Turtles, and Other Hand-held Cosmic Models," *Mission Ignition / Reflections of Divinity* (blog), 1991.

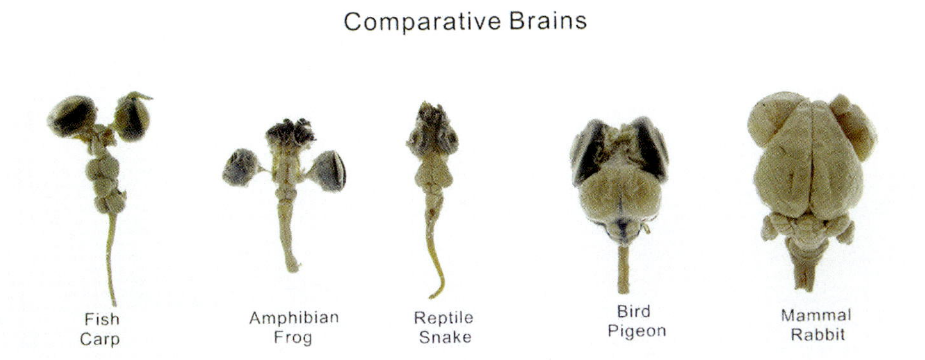

Figure 63. Comparative brains of fish, frog, snake, pigeon and rabbit, suppended in resin block. Purchased at Evolution store in New York City.

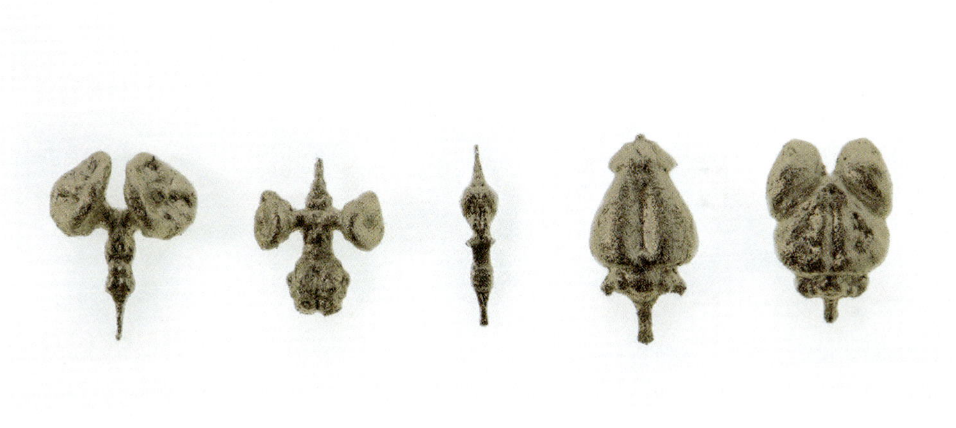

Figure 64. Suzanne Anker, rapid prototype sculptures, modeled after animal brains, 2009. Photograph by Raul Valverde.

encased specimen of animal brains which I had purchased at Evolution, a store which sells natural history "artifacts." Some of my figurines are, in fact, digitally-created images generated from the brain specimens themselves. The presence of Venus figures remains enigmatic to art historians and archaeologists. Most commonly considered as fertility icons, they point to life's interest in reproducing itself.

SF: In art theory there is an ongoing debate about the relation between objects and sculptures. Sculptures are – traditionally – crafted while objects are either found or fabricated. Are the *Biota* pieces objects, sculptures, or both?

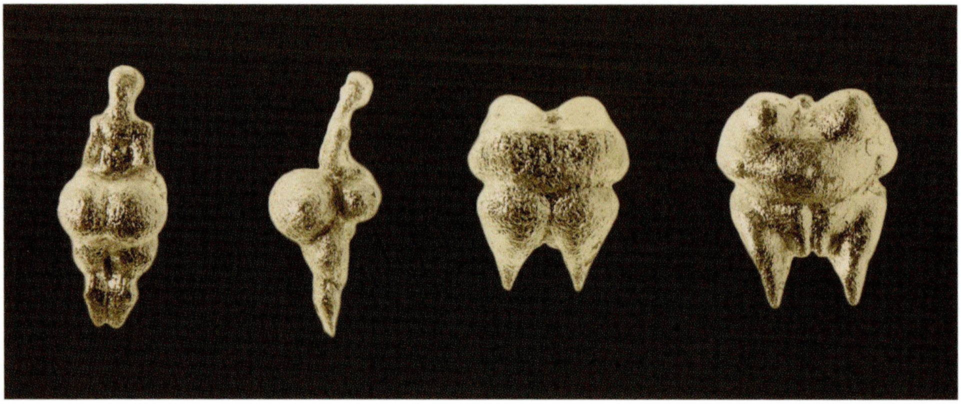

Figure 65. Suzanne Anker, rapid prototype "Venus" figurines modeled after prehistoric originals. Photograph by Raul Valverde.

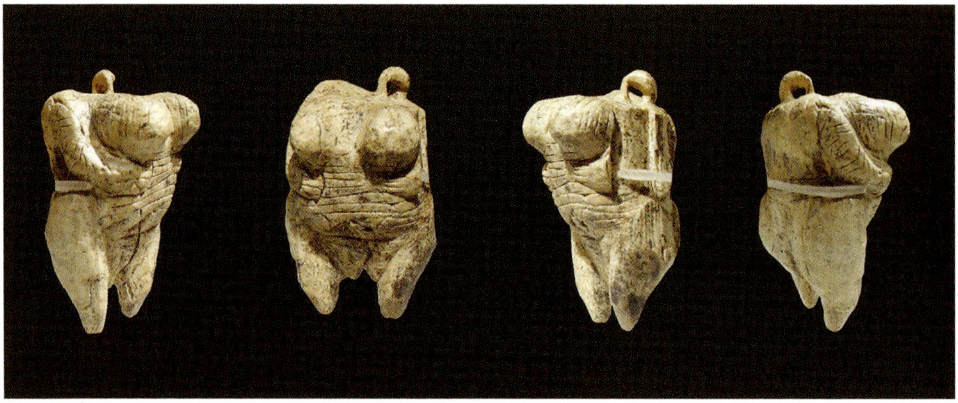

Figure 66. Original Venus from Hohle Fels, mammoth ivory, Aurignacian, aged about 35-40000 years. Discovered in September 2008 in the cave "Hohle Fels" in the Ach Valley near Schelklingen, Germany. Pictures were taken at Urgeschichtliches Museum, Blaubeuren, Germany.

SA: I assume you are referring to Donald Judd's hypothesis concerning *specific objects* and minimalist art.[6] For Judd, metaphor was a condition akin to a microbial infection. The purity of perception and its interception by phenomenology and Gestalt psychology was his mantra. Metaphor was to be eliminated at all costs, heralding in a pure way to physically respond to spatial concerns. However, what he didn't realize is that metaphors do not only refer to narratives or fictions, but are structurally intertwined with our nervous system, language and other com-

6 Donald Judd and Thomas Kellein. *Donald Judd: 1955-1968* (New York: D.A.P., 2002).

munication capabilities.[7] *Biota* is both object and sculpture. The pieces are the residue of a transformation process of a ready-made entity – a natural sea sponge. The original sea sponge disappears through a burnout process to produce what remains, which I refer to as "ghost of sponge." Perhaps that is a new category, when the initial object does in fact disappear.

Curator Deiter Buchhart organized an exhibition at the Marianne Boesky Gallery in New York City entitled *The Nature of Disappearance*[8] in the summer of 2012. The exhibition was held in two locations, one uptown and the other downtown. Buchhart's thesis concerning the exhibition "explores the *nature of disappearance*, that is, the concept of the literal, physical loss of the artwork and in doing so further analyzes how artists who have come after Strindberg and Munch not only question the intactness of the object and the artwork but also literally allow nature to create the work and challenge material integrity, ultimately annihilating the art object."[9] Artists featured in the show included Lucio Fontana, Félix González-Torres, Hermann Nitsch, Gina Pane, and Dieter Roth.

SF: What are the references for your piece entitled *Collision of the Diamond Mind*? Why did you choose this title?

SA: This piece is actually an extension of an earlier work entitled *Diamond-Cutters*, an installation from 1978.[10] The former installation employed limestone, handmade paper, plaster, chalk and broken glass. All of the pieces were white, some of the stones were cut, while others had the residue of dynamite marks left from the stone's extraction from its quarry. The theme of diamond mind is an invocation of clarity and centeredness held by Buddhist philosophers. As a path towards a more enlightened being, the experience of art-making converts energy into form.

SF: This work appears as if it was metal, although it is ceramic. Why did you employ a metallic glaze?

SA: The metallic glaze brings into focus another metaphor: the pieces reference meteorites, which originate from outer space. They are like falling stars. Many of the particles from outer space create debris fields when they encounter earth.

---

7 Raymond W. Gibbs, "The Neural Theory of Metaphor," *The Cambridge Handbook of Metaphor and Thought* (New York: Cambridge University Press, 2008), 17.

8 The catalog of the exhibition was published by Marianne Boesky Gallery in 2014.

9 Exhibition press release.

10 This installation was presented at the Terry Moore Gallery in Saint Louis, Missouri. Art historian and curator Sidra Stich reviewed the exhibition of the *Diamond-Cutter's* series for the The New Art Examiner, March 1978, vol. 5, no. 6.

Collision of the Diamond Mind, points to how little we know about outer space and the imaginary dreams that may be located there. This piece also invokes aspects of chance and flux and how such collisions are beyond our control. *Collision of the Diamond Mind* is, in a sense, an oxymoron. Like *The Glass Veil,* which brings together oppositions, this series of work enjoins concentrated stillness with random forcefulness.

References

Association for International Cancer Research. "Sea Sponges: Tweak of Nature in Fight Against Cancer." ScienceDaily. www.sciencedaily.com/releases/2011/02/110218083600.htm.

Bruno, M. A., F. Pellas, and S. Laureys. "Quality of Life in Locked-in Syndrome Survivors." In *Yearbook of Intensive Care and Emergency Medicine 2008*, edited by J. L Vincent, 881-890. Berlin: Springer, 2008.

Buchhart, Dieter. *The Nature of Disappearance*. New York: Marianne Boesky Gallery, 2014.

Dickinson, Emily. *The Complete Poems of Emily Dickinson*. Boston, Mass: Little, Brown, 1960.

Dumas, Alexandre. *The Count of Monte Cristo*. New York: Modern Library, 1996.

Gibbs, Raymond W. "The Neural Theory of Metaphor." In *The Cambridge Handbook of Metaphor and Thought*, 17-38 . New York: Cambridge University Press, 2008.

Hagens, Bethe. "Venuses, Turtles, and Other Hand-held Cosmic Models." *Mission Ignition / Reflections of Divinity* (blog). 1991. http://missionignition.net/bethe/venus_turtles.php.

Judd, Donald, and Thomas Kellein. *Donald Judd: 1955-1968*. New York: D.A.P., 2002.

Sanders, Robert. "Genome of Ancient Sponge Reveals Origins of First Animals, Cancer." *UC Berkeley NewsCenter: News from the University of California, Berkeley* (blog). August 4, 2010. http://newscenter.berkeley.edu/2010/08/04/sponge_genome/.

Stich, Sidra. "Diamond-Cutter's Series." *The New Art Examiner* (Chicago), March, 1978.

Tel Aviv University. "Common Marine Sponges May Provide Super-antibiotics Of The Future." *ScienceDaily*. March 4, 2009. www.sciencedaily.com/releases/2009/02/090226110743.htm.

Zola, Émile. *Thérèse Raquin*. [Paris]: Garnier-Flammarion, 1970.

List of Illustrations

Fig. 58: Suzanne Anker, *Biota*, 2011. Porcelain, rapid prototype figurines with silver-leaf, plexiglass, 48 x 96 x 9 in (122 x 244 x 22.8 cm). Installation view of *Cerebral Spirits: Stalking the Self* at the Ben Shahn Center for the Visual Arts, William Paterson University Galleries, 2012. Photograph by Raul Valverde.

Fig. 59: Suzanne Anker, *Biota*, 2011 (detail). Porcelain, rapid prototype figurines with silver-leaf, plexiglass, 48 x 96 x 9 in (122 x 244 x 22.8 cm). Installation view of *Cerebral Spirits: Stalking the Self* at the Ben Shahn Center for the Visual Arts, William Paterson University Galleries, 2012. Photograph by Raul Valverde.

Fig. 60: Suzanne Anker, *Carbon Collision In the Diamond Mind*, 2013 (detail). Metallic-glazed porcelain, plexiglass. 48 x 96 x 9 in (122 x 244 x 22.8 cm). Installation view of *While Darkness Sleeps* at the McKinney Avenue Contemporary (The MAC), Dallas, Texas. Photograph by Fernando Rojas.

Fig. 61: Suzanne Anker, Metallic-glazed porcelain sculptures from the *Carbon Collision In the Diamond Mind* installation, 2013. Metallic-glazed porcelain. Dimensions (from left to right): Top: 6 x 5 x 3.5 in (15.2 x 12.7 x 8.9 cm); 9 x 6.5 x 4 in (22.8 x 16.5 x 10.1 cm); 8 x 5 x 5 in (20.3 x 12.7 x 12.7 cm); Middle: 9 x 6.5 x 4 in (22.8 x 16.5 x 10.1 cm); 10 x 9.5 x 4 in (25.4 x 24.1 x 10.1 cm); 7.5 x 4 x 4.5 in (19 x 10.1 x 11.4 cm); Bottom: 10 x 9.5 x 5 in (25.4 x 24.1 x 12.7 cm); 7.5 x 6 x 3 in (19 x 15.2 x 7.6 cm); 11 x 9 x 6.5 in (28 x 22.8 x 16.5 cm). Photographs by Raul Valverde.

Fig. 62: Suzanne Anker. *Carbon Collision In the Diamond Mind*, 2013 (detail). Metallic-glazed porcelain, plexiglass, 48 x 96 x 9 in (122 x 244 x 22.8 cm). Installation view of *FotoFest: Remote Sensing: Microlandscapes and Untold Stories* at Deborah Colton Gallery, Houston, Texas, 2014. Photograph by Henry G. Sanchez.

Fig. 63: Comparative brains of fish, frog, snake, pigeon and rabbit, suspended in resin block. Purchased at Evolution store in New York City.

Fig. 64: Suzanne Anker, Silver-leaf rapid propotype sculptures modeled after animal brains, 2009. Photograph by Raul Valverde.

Fig. 65: Suzanne Anker, silver-leaf papid prototype venus figurines modeled after prehistoric originals. Photograph by Raul Valverde.

Fig. 66: Original Venus from Hohle Fels, mammoth ivory, Aurignacian, aged about 35-40000 years. Discovered in September 2008 in the cave "Hohler Fels" in the Ach Valley near Schelklingen, Germany. Pictures were taken at Urgeschichtliches Museum, Blaubeuren, Germany.

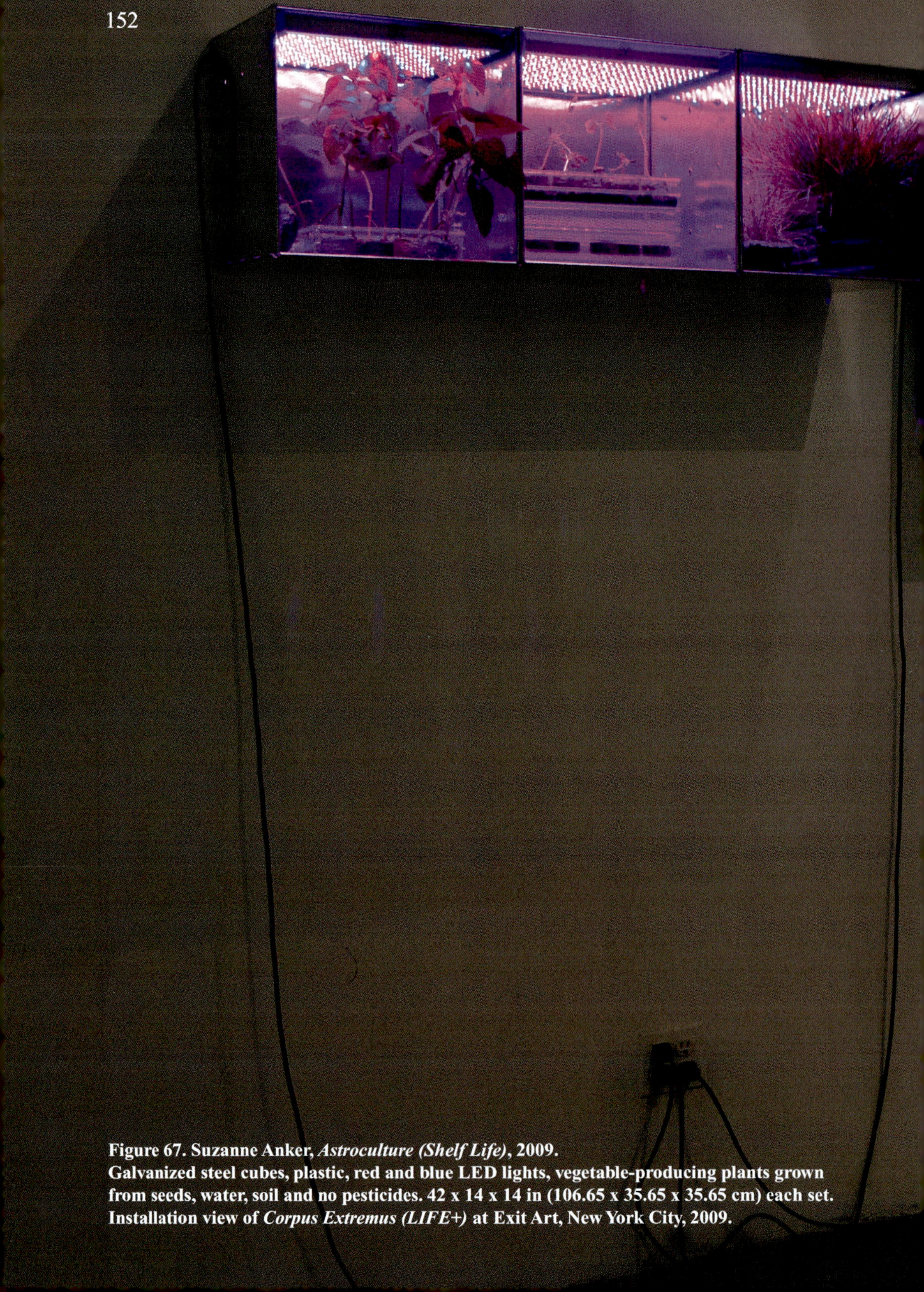

Figure 67. Suzanne Anker, *Astroculture (Shelf Life)*, 2009.
Galvanized steel cubes, plastic, red and blue LED lights, vegetable-producing plants grown from seeds, water, soil and no pesticides. 42 x 14 x 14 in (106.65 x 35.65 x 35.65 cm) each set. Installation view of *Corpus Extremus (LIFE+)* at Exit Art, New York City, 2009.

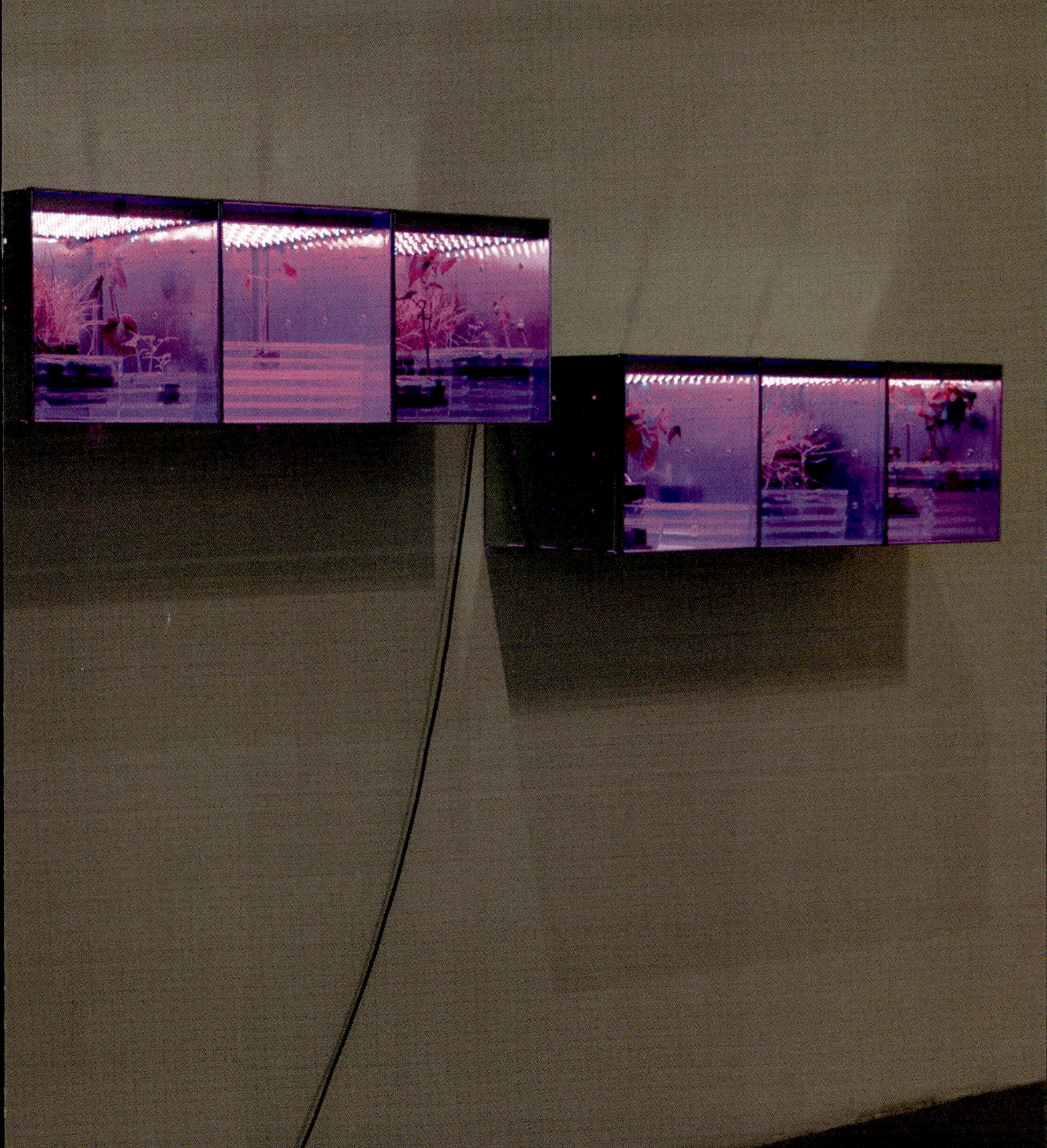

Dialogue VI: Astroculture (Shelf Life)

SUZANNE ANKER & SABINE FLACH

Sabine Flach: *Astroculture (Shelf Life)* (figs. 67-71) is an artwork consisting of photographs, living plants, metal cubes and LED lights. What is the genesis of this piece?

Suzanne Anker: This sculpture is an indoor vegetable and herb garden, created for the exhibition *Corpus Extremus (Life+)*, curated by Boryana Rossa as part of Exit Art's Curatorial Program in 2009. It is similar to both a terrarium and a *Wunderkammer* but also relates to NASA's ongoing Space program. With the rise of biotechnologies and tinkering of living systems, can we imagine what vast resources are still available in outer space and deep sea habitats? How do plants respond to changes in gravity? What happens to seeds, for example, when they are grown in space? NASA's *Space Product Development Program* is exploring these possibilities. The first growth facility installed in 2001 at the International Space Station was aptly named Advanced Astroculture™.[1]

In my work *Astroculture (Shelf Life),* three plant chambers were constructed from off-the-shelf components. Each set consisted of galvanized metal cubes with an inset LED panel. Placed inside the cubes were plastic dishes supporting peat pods implanted with vegetable seeds. Like Russian dolls, there is an internal stacking at play which maintains optimum environmental conditions. Over a period of days the plants began to sprout, forming vines, leaves and flowers, and finally string beans and peas. There were no insecticides employed, and the plants were watered on a regular basis. Surprisingly, although the plants appeared to be fuchsia-colored, they were, in fact, green. The glowing LEDs electrified the space while manifesting the possibility of growing herbs even in any New York City light-deprived apartment. One can say these fuchsia radiances are in masquerade as they herald in the "new green," complete with low carbon footprints and exempt from poisonous chemical agents.

SF: The American photographer Edward Steichen used plants in his work (fig. 72). He compared his activities of breeding and grafting plants to making photographs. Do you see a connection to Steichen in your work?

1 Zhou et al., "Performance of the Advanced ASTROCULTURE Plant Growth Unit During ISS-6A/7A Mission," *SAE Technical Paper,* July 7, 2002.

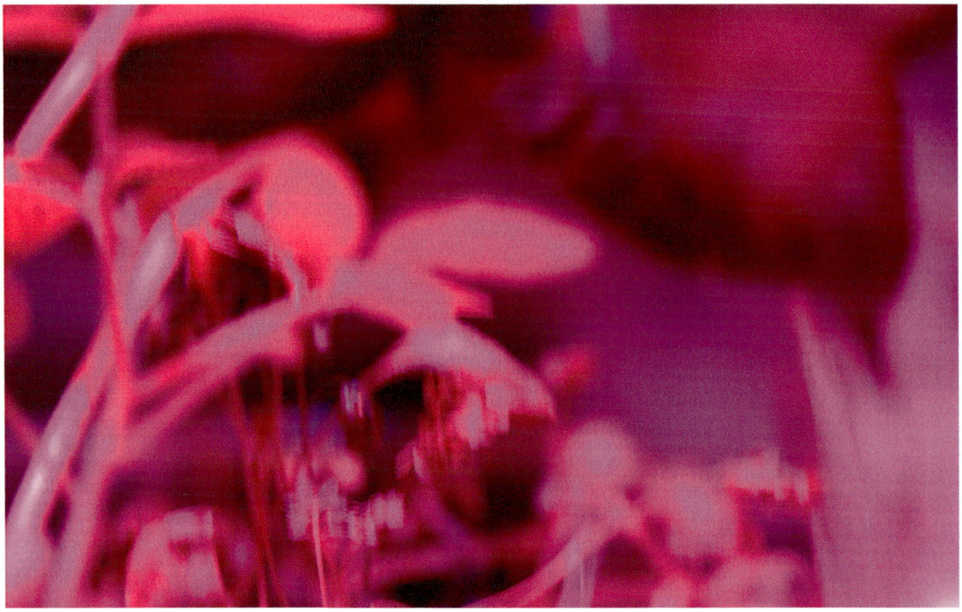

Figure 68. Suzanne Anker, *Astroculture (Shelf Life) #12*, 2009.
Archival inkjet print on paper, 24 x 36 in (60.9 x 91.4 cm).

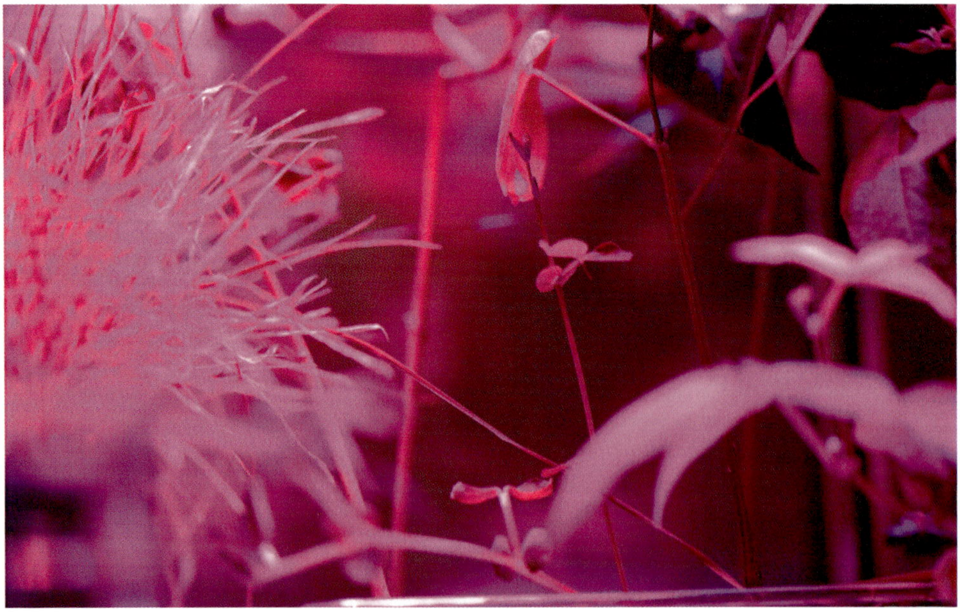

Figure 69. Suzanne Anker, *Astroculture (Shelf Life) #17*, 2009.
Archival inkjet print on paper, 24 x 36 in (60.9 x 91.4 cm).

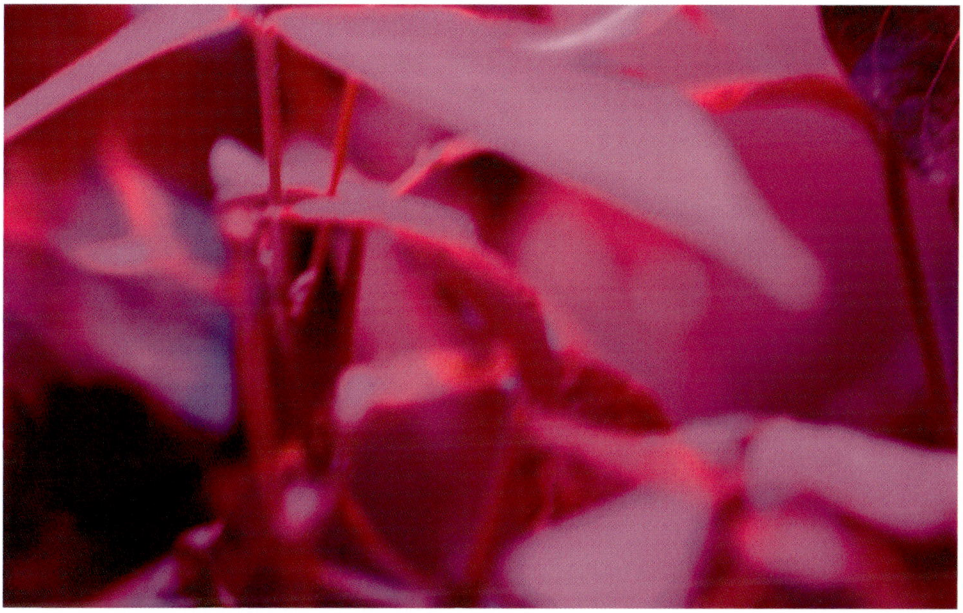

Figure 70. Suzanne Anker, *Astroculture (Shelf Life) #13*, 2009.
Archival inkjet print on paper, 24 x 36 in (60.9 x 91.4 cm).

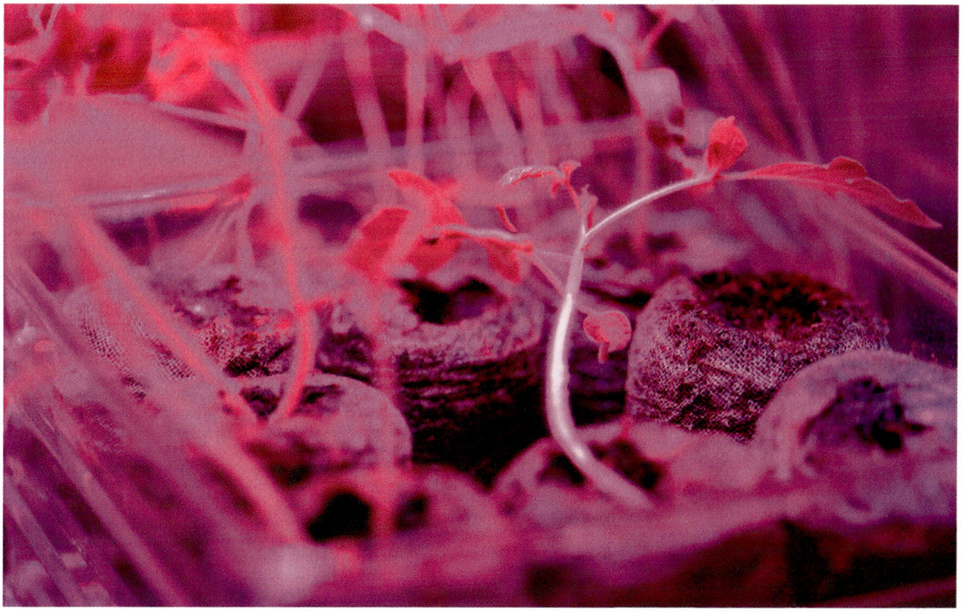

Figure 71. Suzanne Anker, *Astroculture (Shelf Life) #18*, 2009.
Archival inkjet print on paper, 24 x 36 in (60.9 x 91.4 cm).

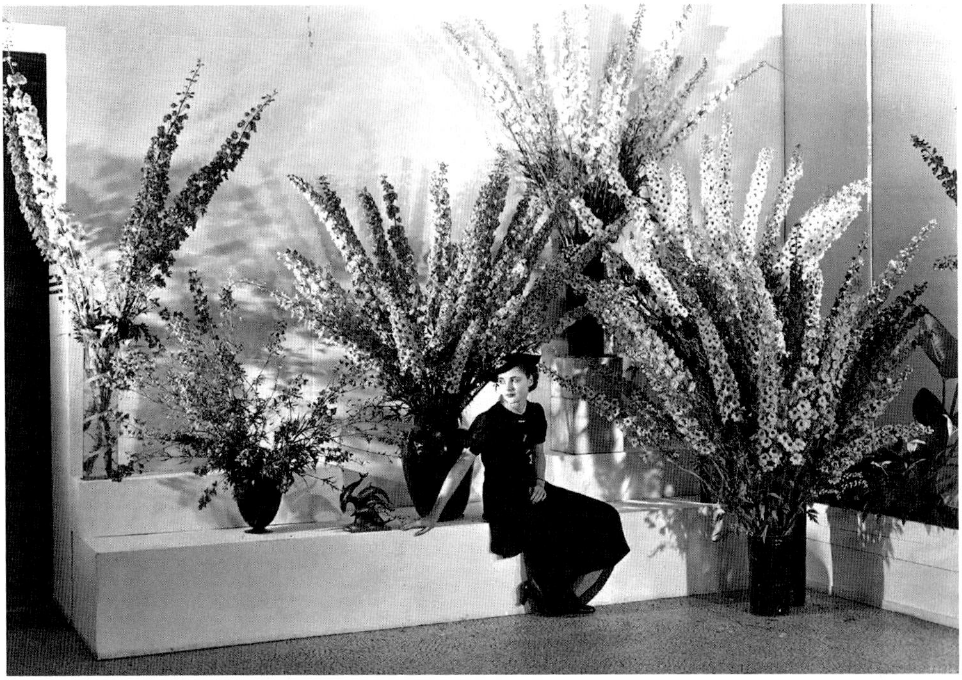

Figure 72. Installation view of the exhibition *Edward Steichen's Delphiniums*. June 24, 1936 through July 1, 1936. The Museum of Modern Art, New York. Photograph by Edward Steichen. © 2014 The Estate of Edward Steichen / Artists Rights Society (ARS), New York. © The Museum of Modern Art/Licensed by SCALA / Art Resource, NY

SA: Steichen was a man of many talents, from museum professional to photographer to horticulturist. He was the first artist to have his delphiniums, a species of flower, exhibited in the Museum of Modern Art in New York City in 1936. He worked with these flowers on ten acres of his 400-acre estate in Connecticut. He employed a chemical mutagen called colchicine, a compound to treat gout in humans, as a device to alter the chromosomal number of the flowers. This chemical substance doubled the number of chromosomes in the plant's chloroplast, which produced six-foot-tall delphiniums in various colors. Touted by some as the father of Bio Art, he remains, with Alexander Fleming[2] before him and his early bacteria paintings, as someone absorbed by the wonders of nature.

SF: In your photographs of *Laboratory Life*, you employed Photoshop software as a way to achieve a simulated double exposure. What digital tools did you employ to achieve such rich painterly effects in *Astroculture (Shelf Life)*?

2 See fig. 97, p. 194 for an example of Fleming's bacterial paintings.

SA: Ironically, these photographs have not been manipulated at all. The large-scale photographs produced in conjunction with this living artwork, were saturated in fluid color as a result of the light available in situ. No Photoshop technology was used. Capturing "liquid light" in this ethereal form produced a set of glowing illusions, exceedingly vibrant and luminescent.

SF: How is your project different from NASA's?

SA: That's a joke, isn't it? NASA's plants are grown in anti-gravity situations and therefore behave differently. Gravity is a force on earth that keeps us from falling off the planet. Our reactions to this pressure are hard-wired into our corporeal selves on earth. Like bodily processes that remain unconscious, our body's counterbalance to gravity is something we take for granted. Antigravitational forces produce various anomalies, for example boiling water in space creates one huge bubble, as opposed to the numerous tiny ones on earth. Flames in outer space are circular, E. coli grow faster, roses smell differently and most relevant here is the way in which vegetable seeds sprout[3]. Japanese astronaut Satoshi Furukawa grew cucumbers in space as part of his space trek. In relation to seed sprouting, what he found was that "on the ground only one peg is made at the time of germination, but under microgravity two pegs were made at the time of sprouting."[4] His specific research delves into the plant hormone auxin, which controls plant growth. What is extraordinary is that everything we know about botany is alternatively refigured in outer space.

SF: Are there other differences in the way plants react?

SA: According to this NASA project, "In microgravity, roots grow latterly [sic] or sideways, instead of up and down like they do under Earth's gravitational forces. Using cucumber plants (scientific name *Cucumis sativus*), investigators look to determine whether hydrotropic – plant root orientation due to water – response can control the direction of root growth in microgravity."[5] Such experimentation challenges our accepted agricultural practices which may be significantly altered depending on environmental circumstances and artificial conditions.

SF: From a philosophical perspective, plants were considered inferior to animals, even in Classical times. In what ways do you acknowledge this difference?

3 Natalie Wolchover, "7 Everyday Things that Happen Strangely In Space." *LiveScience.com*. March 3, 2011.

4 *Space.com*, "Green Thumb in Space: Astronaut to Grow Cosmic Cucumbers." June 7, 2011.

5 Jessica Nimon, "Gardening in Space with HydroTropi." *NASA*. January 14, 2011.

SA: Most plants, as opposed to animals, cannot easily engage in locomotion as they are fixed to the ground. However, they do have quite remarkable sensitivities. They can recognize daughter plants as being connected to them. They have strong reactions to foes and even change their internal rhythms to compensate for dangerous predators. For some theorists, they are like animals, only much slower. Several remarkable films exist which explicate this issue. The first is based on a 1973 text, *The Secret Life of Plants*, written by Peter Tompkins and Christopher Bird. The documentary film of the same name excerpts film footage from Jagadish Chandra Bose's laboratory. Bose, a Bengali physicist, biologist and writer of science fiction, viewed plants as both sentient beings and as potential electrical energy sources.

Another more recent film, hosted by PBS entitled *What Plants Talk About* (2013), follows up on some of the aspects of plant intelligence explored in the earlier film. Experimental plant ecologist, James Cahill, a professor at the University of Alberta, talks about a plant's ability to actively respond to environmental changes. Although plants have no brain, eyes or ears, they can still communicate.

SF: There have been discussions about plant phenomenology, a sub-genre of this profound philosophical discipline being given over to vegetal life. What does this sub-discipline propose as an extension of phenomenology?

SA: In Michael Marder's *Plant Thinking: A Philosophy of Vegetal Life,* the author talks about plant thinking as a non-cognitive and non-imagistic mode of thinking. In part, his text is a reaction to the mounting research in cultural studies centered around the "animal." He views "plants as our non-human others". Although they are sensile, they are not passive. He rests his assertion on the phenomenological concept of intentionality. For the philosopher, his aim is to "rethink concepts such as being-sensile and being-in-a-place" as well as "how above ground and underground environments appear to plants."[6] These are empirical experiences we, as humans, cannot fathom. He quotes Immanuel Kant's *Critique of Judgment*, in this regard: "It is utterly impossible for human reason [...] to hope to understand the generation even of a blade of grass from mere mechanical causes." Such awe and reverence for living things is ultimately inspiring.

SF: What other work have you done with plants?

SA: I have worked with African violets as a model organism for performing tissue culturing experiments. Beginning with a piece of leaf or stem – a sliver of a

6 Michael Marder, "Plant intentionality and the phenomenological framework of plant intelligence." *Plant Signaling & Behavior* 7, no. 11 (2012): 1365-1372.

plant–these fragments are put into small glass jars containing agar, plant hormones, nutrients and antibiotics. These initial bits are called explants. The sterile container is then sealed and placed under a light source which is activated by a timer. This on-again, off-again scenario allows for equal time of radiant light and complete darkness. When the explants begin to mature and become microplants, they are then separated and replanted into new jars. This is repeated again until the plants outgrow their jars. They are then acclimated into soil and continue to grow. As they mature they are transferred into pots where they develop larger leaves and finally bloom. Each plant is identical from a molecular point of view, yet individual plants look slightly different from their siblings and adapt to the environment in slightly divergent ways.

SF: How do you account for this? Isn't a clone an exact copy?

SA: There are no exact copies produced by nature. Even identical twins have fingerprints at variance. This experiment drives home the point that epigenetics is an area that requires comprehensive study. How the environment, even on a micro scale, transforms gene sequences? While this concept has become more widely researched since the decipherment of the human genome, early investigations into this phenomenon were formulated by the erudite British biologist C. H. Waddington. He termed these molecular actions in metaphorical language, coining the term "epigenetic landscape," as an explanation for gene regulation and expression.

SF: Recently you reconstructed *Astroculture (Shelf Life)* in Berlin at Art Laboratory (2014). How was this installation different from the one at Exit Art?

SA: My installation at Exit Art in New York City consisted of a completely dark space. On one side of my piece was Australian performance artists Stelarc's video of his "third ear" surgery and on the other side was a backlit piece by Oron Catts, a tableau of taxidermied animals and his tissue culture machine. I had assumed incorrectly that ambient light would not interfere with how the piece could be photographed. However, after photographing *Astroculture (Shelf Life)* at Art Laboratory Berlin (figs. 73, 74), the images radiated a blue presence. I attribute this to the fact that the gallery space has a front window which let in daylight.

SF: What future projects do you have with plants?

SA: I love plants. I love their regenerative properties, particularly perennials, especially in spring when the first flowering bulbs begin to sprout and the tree buds make their presence known as they get ready to burst open. This renewal makes me think of nature's developmental cycle and its capacity for rebounding.

I am currently working with Sebastian Cocioba, a botanist who has cloned over 100,000 orchids. His company, NY Botanics is a small startup that he individually runs. We are working together on an experimental synthetic biology project. We are obtaining the hereditary material from two distinct plants and attempting to fuse them together with the intention of producing a third variety. There are many technical issues involved in this procedure as plant sterility may be induced, negating the production of seeds. According to Cocioba: "Traditional plant breeding uses pollen as the vehicle for change. The pollen carries the traits of one plant and mixes, via sexual reproduction, with the egg cells of another plant, thus producing offspring which are hybrids of the two parent plants. This process is very well established and has been utilized for millennia, but is limited to plants within the same species. We plan to take the concept of genetic mixing and produce a novel hybrid by crossing plants that would otherwise be impossible to generate by traditional means. In its simplest form, we will take leaf tissue from each plant and strip them down to a puree of free cells and then force said cells to fuse like soap bubbles using chemicals that bring particles together. The fused cells will be a perfect mix, genetically, of the two different plants and will be regenerated into a complete mature plant expressing, theoretically, the characteristics of both parents. Since the combination will be a genetic mix, there is a good chance of producing new and never before seen physical traits which include, but are not limited to, color, shape, floral aroma, growth patterns, etc."[7] This is a complex and time-consuming project in which outcomes are unknown. Although this might be a complete failure, it is with blind determination that we proceed. This project is named *Synthetic Abandon*, after a text I wrote in 1992, which appears in the Appendix of this volume (page 211). This text speaks of obsessions, which adequately describe the repetitions, permutations and high- stake pleasures achieved by realizations of discovery.

7 Email correspondence.

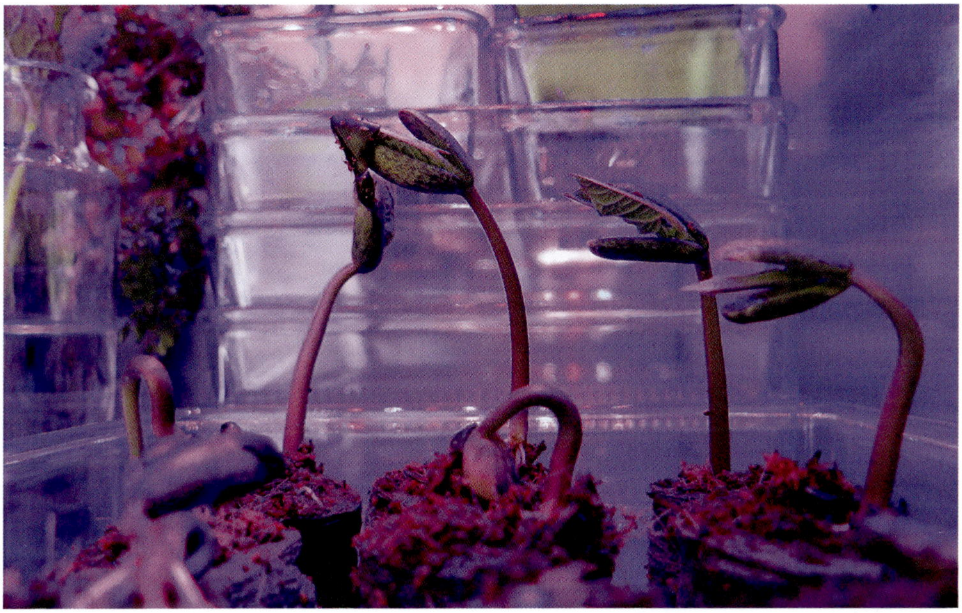

Figure 73. Suzanne Anker, *Astroculture (Shelf Life) II*, 2014. Installation view of *[macro]biologies II: organisms*, at Art Laboratory, Berlin, 2014. Photograph by Suzanne Anker.

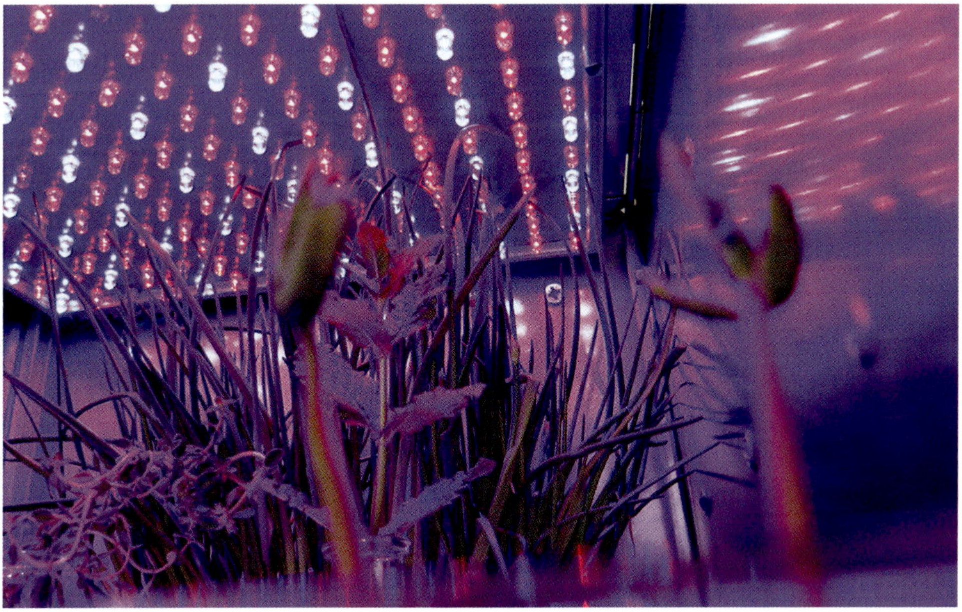

Figure 74. Suzanne Anker, *Astroculture (Shelf Life) II*, 2014. Installation view of *[macro]biologies II: organisms*, at Art Laboratory, Berlin, 2014. Photograph by Suzanne Anker.

References

Dunn, Rob. "Painting With Penicillin: Alexander Fleming's Germ Art." *Smithsonian Magazine online* (blog). July, 2011. http://www.smithsonianmag.com/science-nature/painting-with-penicillin-alexander-flemings-germ-art-1761496.

Goldberg, Aaron D., C. D. Allis, and Emily Bernstein. "Epigenetics: A Landscape Takes Shape." *Cell* 128, no. 4 (2007): 635-638. doi:10.1016/j.cell.2007.02.006.

Hartmann, Celia. "Edward Steichen Archive: Delphiniums Blue (and White and Pink, Too)." *MoMA / Museum of Modern Art* (blog). March 8, 2011. http://www.moma.org/explore/inside_out/2011/03/08/edward-steichen-archive-delphiniums-blue-and-white-and-pink-too.

Marder, Michael. *Plant-Thinking: A Philosophy of Vegetal Life*. New York: Columbia University Press, 2013.

Marder, Michael. "Plant intentionality and the phenomenological framework of plant intelligence." *Plant Signaling & Behavior* 7, no. 11 (2012): 1365-1372. doi:10.4161/psb.21954.

Nature: What Plants Talk About. Directed by Erna Buffie. 2013. Arlington, Virginia: Public Broadcasting Service (PBS), DVD.

Nimon, Jessica. "Gardening in Space with HydroTropi." *NASA* (blog). January 14, 2011. http://www.nasa.gov/mission_pages/station/research/news/hydrotropi.html.

Space.com (blog). "Green Thumb in Space: Astronaut to Grow Cosmic Cucumbers." June 7, 2011. http://www.space.com/11887-space-station-astronaut-grows-cucumbers.html.

Waddington, Conrad H. *Organisers and Genes*. Cambridge: Cambridge University Press, 1940

Wolchover, Natalie. "7 Everyday Things that Happen Strangely In Space." *LiveScience.com* (blog). March 3, 2011. http://www.livescience.com/33091-slideshow-strange-everyday-things-space.html.

Zhou, W., S.J. Durst, M. DeMars, B. Stankovic, B.M. Link, G. Tellez, R.A. Meyers, P.W. Sandstrom, and J.R. Abba. "Performance of the Advanced ASTROCULTURE Plant Growth Unit During ISS-6A/7A Mission." *SAE Technical Papers* (blog). July 7, 2002. http://papers.sae.org/2002-01-2280/.

List of Illustrations

Fig. 67: Suzanne Anker, *Astroculture (Shelf Life)*, 2009. Galvanized steel cubess, plastic, red & blue LED lights, plants, water, soil and no pesticides. 14 x 14 x 14 in (35.65 x 35.65 x 35.65 cm). Vegetable producing plants grown from seed using LED lights. Installation view of *Corpus Extremus (LIFE+)* at Exit Art, NYC, 2009.
Fig. 68: Suzanne Anker, *Astroculture (Shelf Life) #12*, 2009. Archival inkjet print on paper, 24 x 36 in (60.9 x 91.4 cm).
Fig. 69: Suzanne Anker, *Astroculture (Shelf Life) #17*, 2009. Archival inkjet print on paper, 24 x 36 in (60.9 x 91.4 cm).
Fig. 70: Suzanne Anker, *Astroculture (Shelf Life) #13*, 2009. Archival inkjet print on paper, 24 x 36 in (60.9 x 91.4 cm).
Fig. 71: Suzanne Anker, *Astroculture (Shelf Life) #18*, 2009. Archival inkjet print on paper, 24 x 36 in (60.9 x 91.4 cm).
Fig. 72. Installation view of the exhibition, *Edward Steichen's Delphiniums*. June 24, 1936 through July 1, 1936. The Museum of Modern Art, New York. Photograph by Edward Steichen: © 2014 The Estate of Edward Steichen / Artists Rights Society (ARS), New York. © The Museum of Modern Art/Licensed by SCALA / Art Resource, NY.
Fig. 73: Suzanne Anker, *Astroculture (Shelf Life) II*, 2014. Installation view of *[macro]biologies II: organisms*, at Art Laboratory, Berlin, 2014. Photograph by Suzanne Anker.
Fig. 74: Suzanne Anker, *Astroculture (Shelf Life) II*, 2014. Installation view of *[macro]biologies II: organisms*, at Art Laboratory, Berlin, 2014. Photograph by Suzanne Anker.

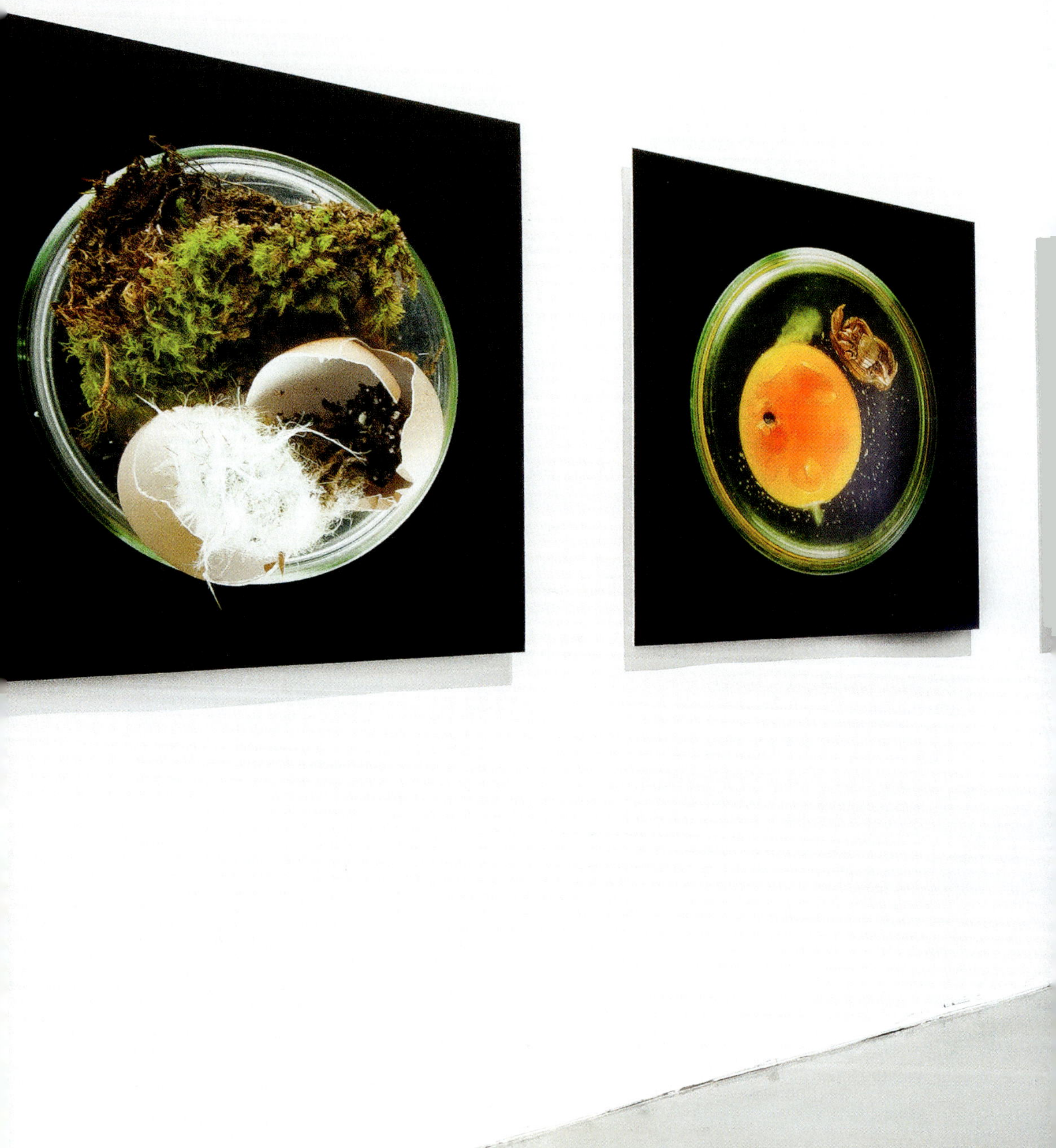

Figure 75. Suzanne Anker, *Vanitas (in a Petri Dish)* series, 2013. Inkjet prints on paper mounted on board, 42 x 42 in (107 x 107 cm) each. Installation view of *Rainbow Loom* at V Art Center, M50 Creative Garden Shanghai, China, 2014. Photograph by Henry G. Sanchez.

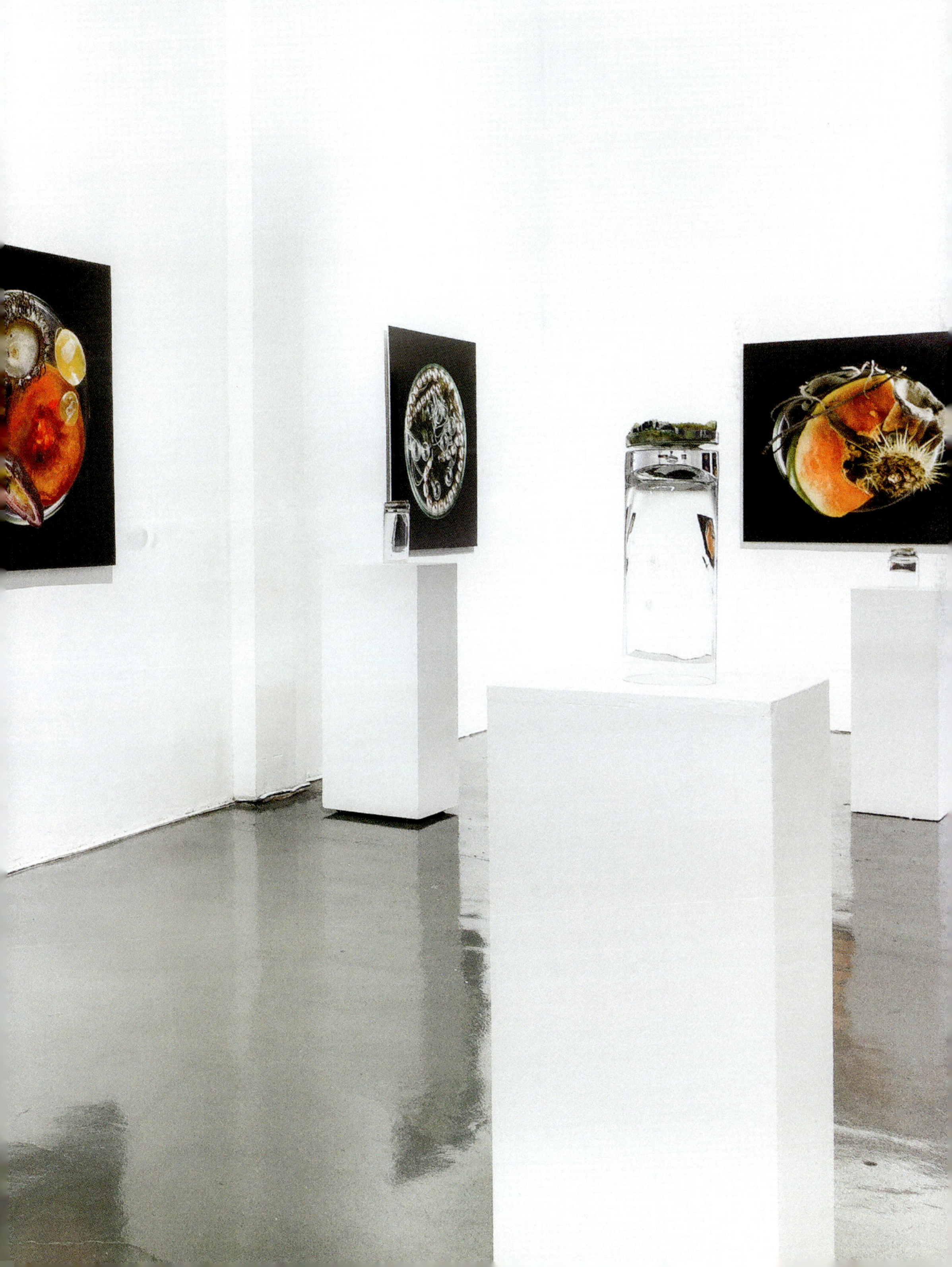

Dialogue VII: Vanitas (in a Petri Dish) / Remote Sensing

SUZANNE ANKER & SABINE FLACH

Sabine Flach: With the series *Vanitas (in a Petri Dish)* it seems that for the first time you create compositions from "found objects"–pearls, feathers, flowers and so on–in your work. Could you describe this kind of shift in your use of materials?

Suzanne Anker: Whether found in nature or industrially fabricated, my materials are arranged in small Petri dishes. Like a little *Wunderkammer*, disparate objects from various origins are assembled in one setting. The objects are chosen for specific physical attributes or symbolic value, as they similarly function in historical vanitas paintings. In prior centuries, such paintings warned against the excesses of material culture and its progressive corruption of spiritual values. In *Vanitas (in a Petri Dish)* the viewer is presented with images of dead insects, fruit-stuffs –which will decay–bones, skulls, minerals, fresh and dried flowers, eggs, metals, glass and such. They are some of the robust offerings from the Earth's pantry. As simple warning about the delicacy of life, we pause in front of this array at our own wonder. The arrangements pictured here are reminders of both life's continuum and death's seemingly finality.

In addition, these pieces indirectly reference the expanding field of synthetic biology, a kind of molecular grafting, bringing into existence new forms of life. As Carl Linnaeus' formal taxonomic categories are overturned through genetic engineering, amalgams of variegated species can be combined and reordered. For example, goats make milk containing silkworm fibers, tomatoes are manipulated to carry a flounder gene, and plants are re-engineered to contain their own chemical herbicide. This kind of fusion is hinted at in the choice of my diverse materials, both organic and inorganic, both dead and alive, both edible and poisonous. The material processes of remaking, repairing, restructuring and revamping are the new "calls of the wild" as natural resources are being exploited and tendered.

SF: Is this shift in your work a new topic or a summary of all your interests in the life sciences? Vanitas motifs are by tradition symbols of the transience and volatility of all life. And this frequently suggests a moral component – is this your ambition as well?

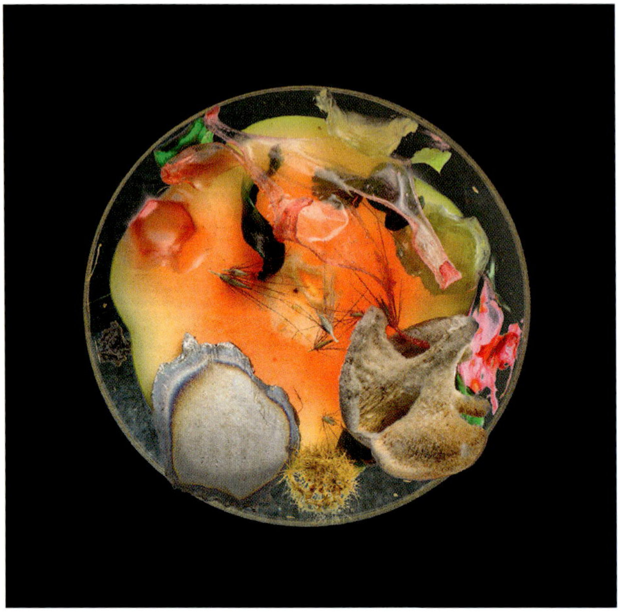

Figure 76. Suzanne Anker, *Vanitas (in a Petri Dish) #8*, 2013.
Archival inkjet print on paper, 42 x 42 in (107 x 107 cm).

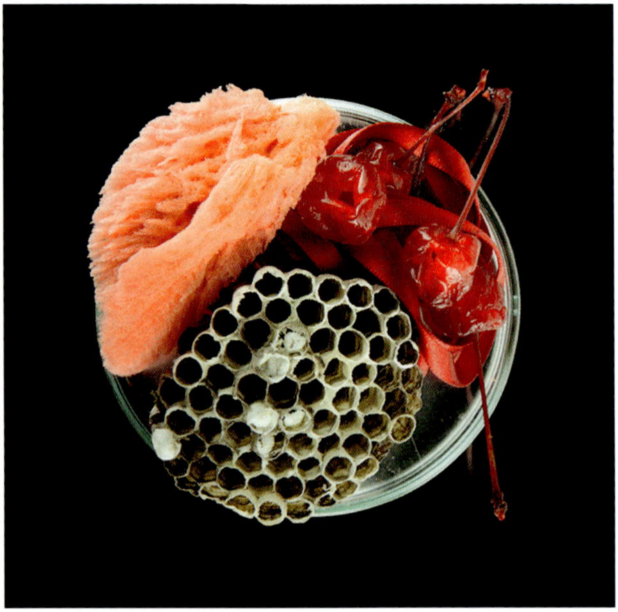

Figure 77. Suzanne Anker, *Vanitas (in a Petri Dish) #3*, 2013.
Archival inkjet print on paper, 42 x 42 in (107 x 107 cm).

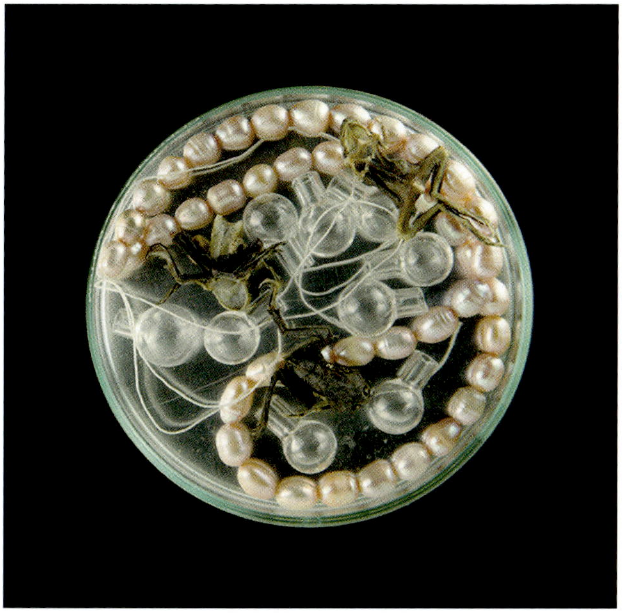

Figure 78. Suzanne Anker, *Vanitas (in a Petri Dish) #2*, 2013.
Archival inkjet print on paper, 42 x 42 in (107 x 107 cm).

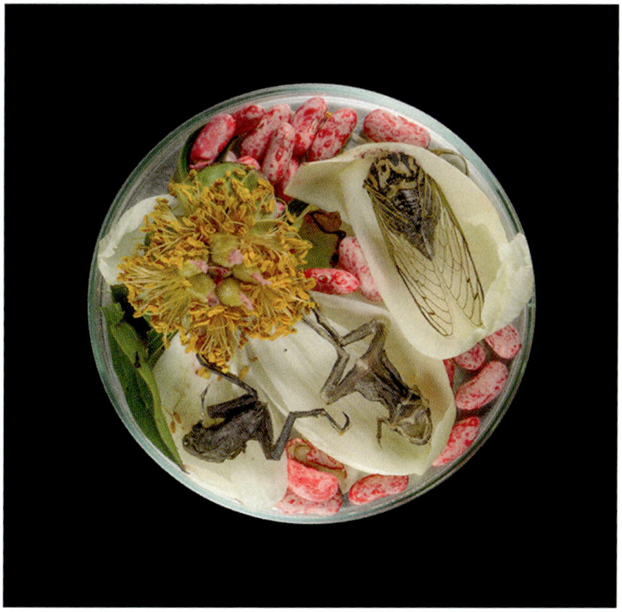

Figure 79. Suzanne Anker, *Vanitas (in a Petri Dish) #15*, 2013.
Archival inkjet print on paper, 42 x 42 in (107 x 107 cm).

SA: The shift in my work is a representation of another level of organic organization. I have been involved with molecules and codes, proteins and chemical signifiers and currently I have moved up the biological ladder to include macro organisms. All living matter does have the common denominator of DNA. In fact, as we ascend the phylogenetic order, we see within ourselves the remnants of our atavistic others: bacteria, ferns, fish, frogs, et al. Manipulations of matter bring with it consequences, warnings if you will, about just how far our mechanistic view of the world has taken us. *Vanitas in a (Petri Dish)* (figs. 76-79, 83, 85), is an update on the 16th-, 17th- and 18th-century visions about these issues.

Vanitas paintings are part of the many images incorporated into art history's still life genre. Meticulously painted as signs of worldly goods, these paintings usually consisted of a mix of elements. From clocks to bones to peeled lemons and candles, from rotting fruit to musical instruments in repose, these images functioned as symbolic warnings against an all too materialistic culture. Moral components of altering nature in the 21st century is a central discourse in bioethics. Since nature is not a fixed entity but combinations of molecules in flux, it is possible currently to mix and match its components.

SF: With the Vanitas motif you are referring to one of the most traditional subjects in art history. Could you please describe the reference to the traditional Vanitas representations in art history? How did that topic come to your interest and why?

SA: From complete makeovers, to *nouveau riche* conceits, the subject of crass materialism has become a modernist deity. Celebrity is a form of religious belief in which followers propose that happiness will follow material success. My images are congruent with the eruption of these kinds of paintings in prior centuries, but my concerns alternatively are secular. Material success may be necessary, but not sufficient in supporting a life well lived.

SF: Vanitas motifs are a highlight during the Baroque era. Another aspect of the Vanitas motif was to confess and to justify its own vanity as an object in the world, as a painting. Is this one of your intentions as well, to critique positions in the art world or art itself?

SA: The art world is a complex "organism" with high drama, as it was in the Baroque era. Its fodder is glittering fame and physical lavishness transposed into art as an index of wealth and status. Art has become an entertainment industry, although there are pockets that support other platforms: art as knowledge production as you have cited, art as social research, art as political exposé, art as transgression, art as an institutional critique. As critic Benjamin Buchloh so elegantly stated in his text *Farewell to an Identity*, "we finally have come to experience the total permeation

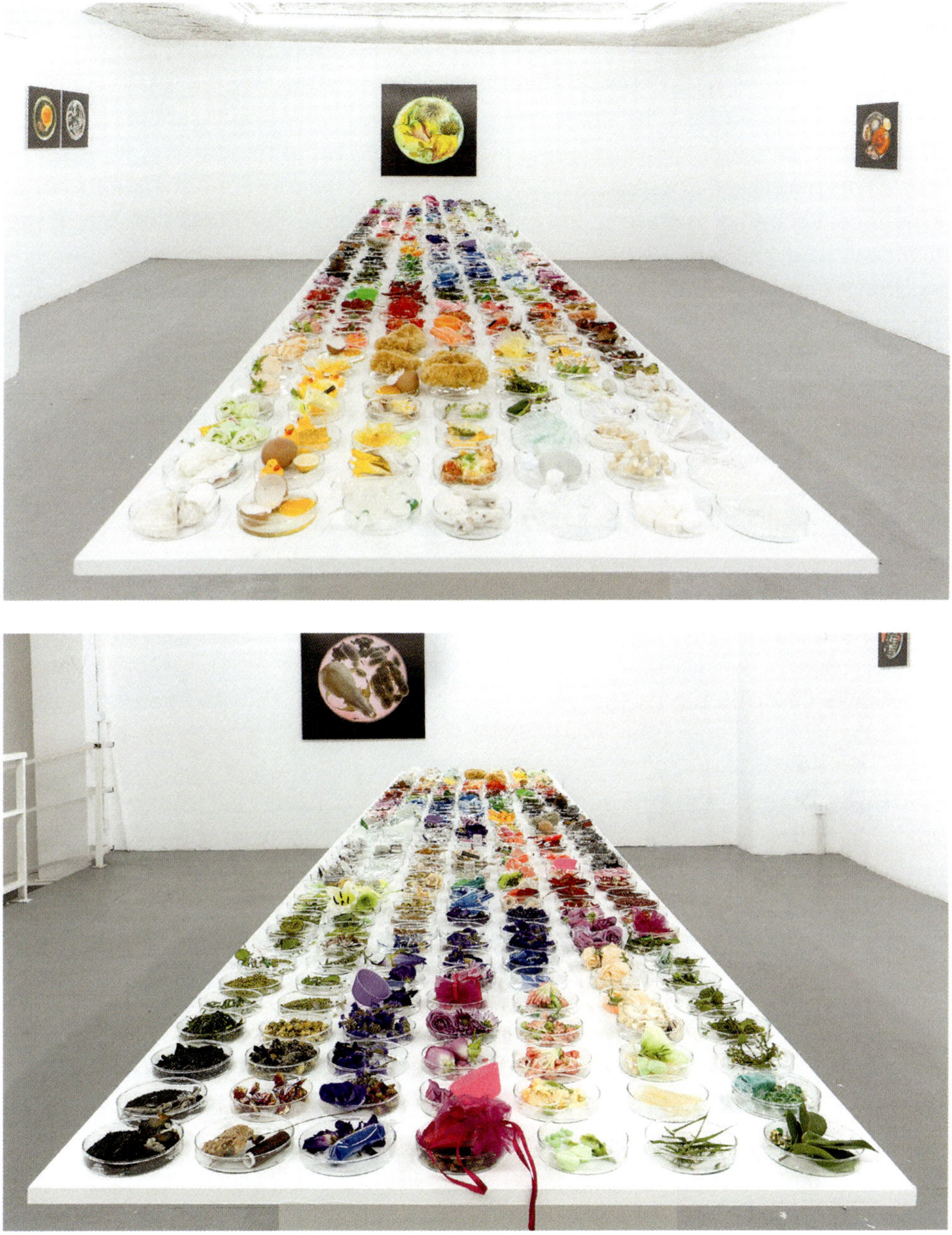

Figure 80. Suzanne Anker, *Rainbow Loom*, 2014.
Wooden table, 366 glass Petri dishes, various items collected in China, 36 x 192 x 36 in (91.4 x 487.7 x 91.4 cm). Installation view of *Rainbow Loom* at V Art Center, M50 Creative Garden Shanghai, China, 2014. Photograph by Henry G. Sanchez.

of the cultural sphere by the economic operations of finance capital and its attendant ethos and social structures."[1] Here he is talking about the final collapse of the avant-garde and its philosophical iterations. He cites Andy Warhol's ironic phrase "business art is the best art" as coming to fruition, *sans* ironic sarcasm. In such an environment spectacle is the main artery grafted on to the art world's artificial heart. This narcissistic corporate ethos has ravaged aspects of culture and its belief structures, such that the largest checkbook holds critical discourse hostage. It has also been said that we live in a time of "the end of nature."[2] Since nature too has become a commodity, everything is fungible. Biology – and its technologies – has migrated into corporate culture as a form of bio-power, and it is no exception to the manner in which the dynamism of endowments articulates their presence.

SF: The presence of absence is a role model for the Vanitas motif: they show the absence of life. Is this paradox something you reflect upon with your work as well?

SA: I wouldn't call it an absence of life but rather life in transition. As organic matter decays it becomes food for other organisms so that a complete cycle or a recycling of molecules and matter takes place. The vanitas in certain ways is a process piece that evokes periodicity and dissolution.

SF: Please describe the relationship between the actual objects you employ and their images as photographs.

SA: Employing digital programs as an interface between existing objects and images requires a significant amount of translation. If we refer to the original set-ups in Petri dishes, which consisted of animal, vegetable and mineral parts, each collection is a "thing itself." When each "still life" was photographed, the image became a stand-in or surrogate for the original materials. Hence, we go from matter to sign, as in all photographic translations.

SF: With the background black or white, The vanitas motifs appear as icons, positioned on black and white background. Icons are the role model for all images. Is this your intention?

SA: I wanted to make a clear distinction between the brightly colored aspects of the piece in relation to the background. The circular image, whether a mandala or tondo, resonates in form with the Petri dish. For me, the Petri dish has become

1 Benjamin H. D. Buchloh, "Farewell to an Identity." *Artforum* 51, no. 4 (2012): 252-263.

2 See Bill McKibben *The End of Nature*.

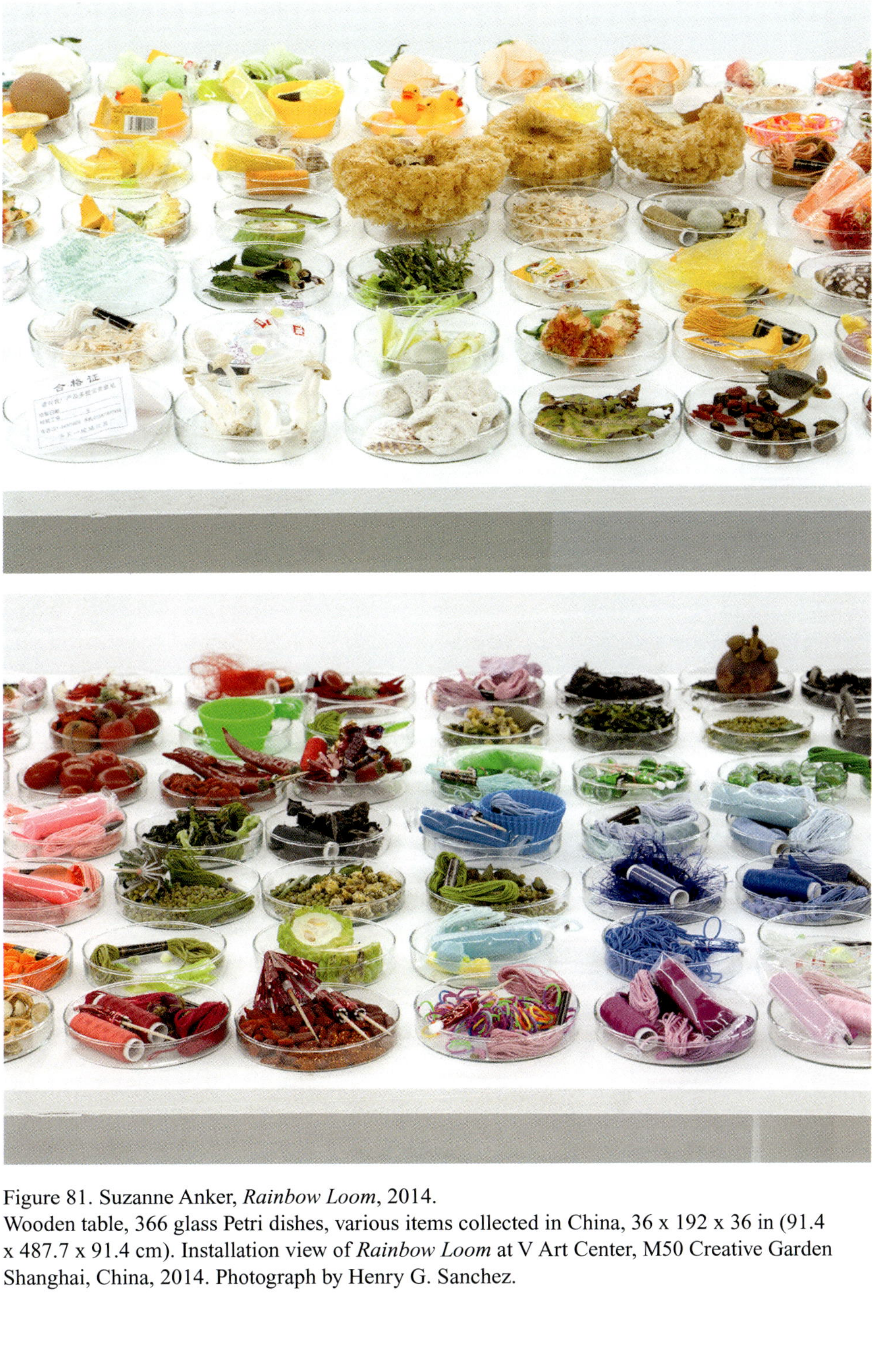

Figure 81. Suzanne Anker, *Rainbow Loom*, 2014.
Wooden table, 366 glass Petri dishes, various items collected in China, 36 x 192 x 36 in (91.4 x 487.7 x 91.4 cm). Installation view of *Rainbow Loom* at V Art Center, M50 Creative Garden Shanghai, China, 2014. Photograph by Henry G. Sanchez.

an icon in itself, representing Bio Art and research science. As a humble glass instrument it has revolutionized scientific discovery, fostering research into microbes and the culturing of cells. Without the Petri dish the ability to proceed with applications designed for in vitro fertilization would be thwarted. This ingenious piece of glassware is, simply, a flat container and a tight fitting lid, engineered to fit under the microscope. It is like another lens in which the changing dynamics of its contents can be viewed. This year I have created two new installations, which employ 200-400 Petri dishes. They posit the Petri dish as a cultural marker, a "ready-made" scientific object recognized by the culture at large. *Petri's Panoply*, named after the German bacteriologist Julius Petri, employs this container as a site for the study of natural objects intermixed with man-made variations, sorted and positioned by color. In Shanghai my exhibition *Rainbow Loom* was composed from articles made in China or found in Chinese markets (fig. 81). In Berlin, all materials were collected on site in Germany (fig. 82).

SF: Can you describe some of the items you arranged in these installations?

SA: The items found in Shanghai included rubber duckies, blue lotus flowers, mushroom varieties, sponge-like fungus, play dough, rubber bands and 1000-year-old eggs, which are sometimes referred to as century-old eggs. When their eggshells are removed, the egg is revealed as a gelatinous mass of black, green and amber. In Berlin, items included broken glass, dead grass hoppers, tomatoes, chicken eggs, steel wool, candy and spices. It is significant to note that, because of international trade, there is an overall uniformity of products however with some exceptions. National identities and class differences are prominently displayed alongside their generic counterparts.

SF: What relationship exists between *Vanitas (in a Petri Dish)* and *Remote Sensing*?

SA: The concept of remote sensing deals with new technologies which can picture places that are either too toxic or difficult to visit. Using state-of-the-art satellite data, remote sensing apparatuses are employed to computationally picture such spaces. As an extension of digital photography, these images garner information electronically in order to eclipse onsite investigations.

The fabrication of *Remote Sensing* begins with the digital photographs *Vanitas (in a Petri Dish)* series. These high-resolution images were reprocessed into a computer program that converts the photographs' brightness into 3D protrusions, a technique called displacement mapping. Next the 3D files were run through software to create a third axis for printing: x, y, and z, the z-axis being coordinate for height. The program also determines the deposition of variegated color applied to the structure as it is being built, one layer at a time. Dark areas were ex-

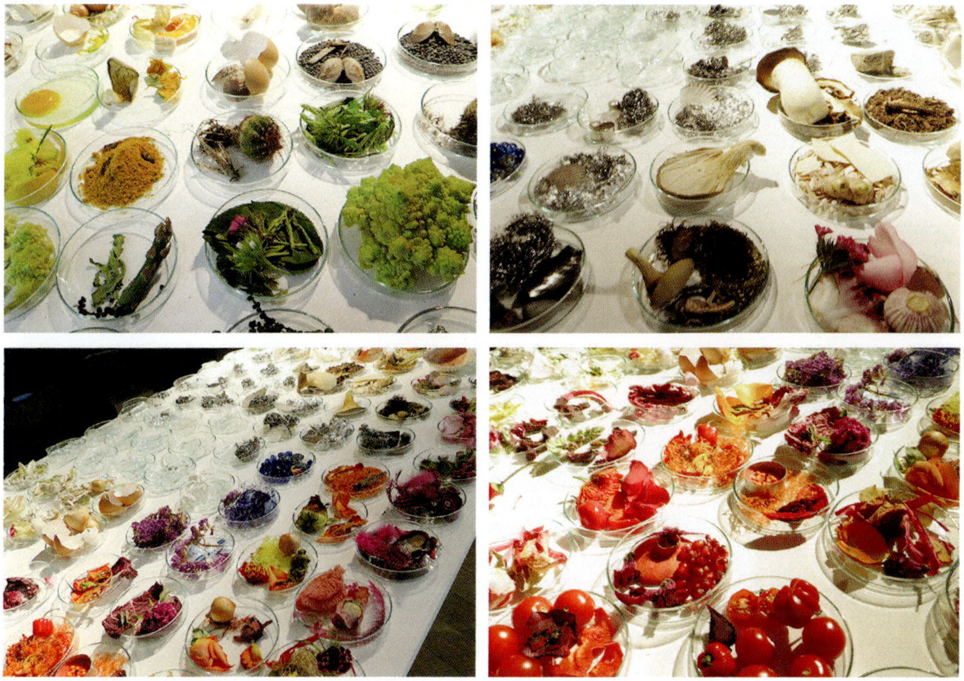

Figure 82. Suzanne Anker, *Petri's Panoply*, 2014. Wooden table, 186 glass Petri dishes, various items collected in Germany, 36 x 96 x 36 in (91.4 x 244 x 91.4 cm). Installation view of *[macro] biologies II: organisms*, Art Laboratory, Berlin, 2014. Photograph by Suzanne Anker.

truded less than bright areas, keeping in tune with the ways which pictorial space visually operates two-dimensionally (figs. 83-86). The resulting objects took on new meaning as a still life became transformed into a microlandscape, ironically, another genre in art historical dialogue. Hence these simulations provide tools for the expansion of pictorial configurations in *both* science and art.

SF: Suzanne, *Vanitas* and *Remote Sensing* (figs. 87-92) in addition to your Petri installations are filled with chromatic intensity. Why did the work become so colorful?

SA: As it turns out, the material world is extremely colorful… full of rich hues and tints. Color entered my work through the incorporation of natural objects and their synthetic others: beads, plastics, threads, fruits, flowers and vegetables along with shells and feathers. The color was already embedded in the objects I was employing. What was so surprising to me was the small amount of blue in the natural world, not including the sea and sky. Lapis lazuli, a beautiful blue stone, has historical significance for painting. Ground into a fine powder, it became a prized pigment for Titian and Vermeer among others.

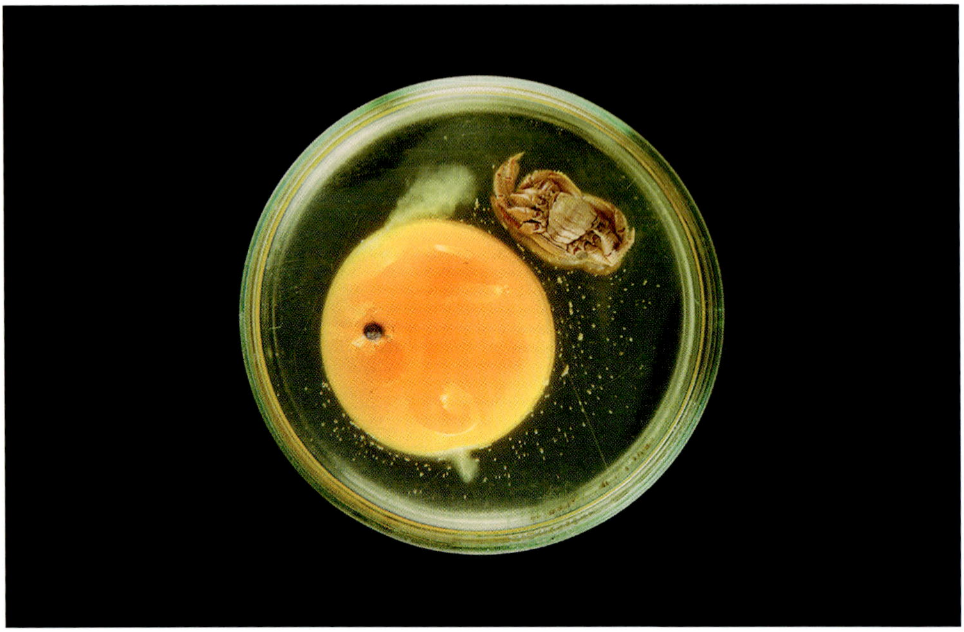

Figure 83. Suzanne Anker, *Vanitas (in a Petri Dish) #1*, 2013.
Archival inkjet print on paper, 42 x 42 in (107 x 107 cm).

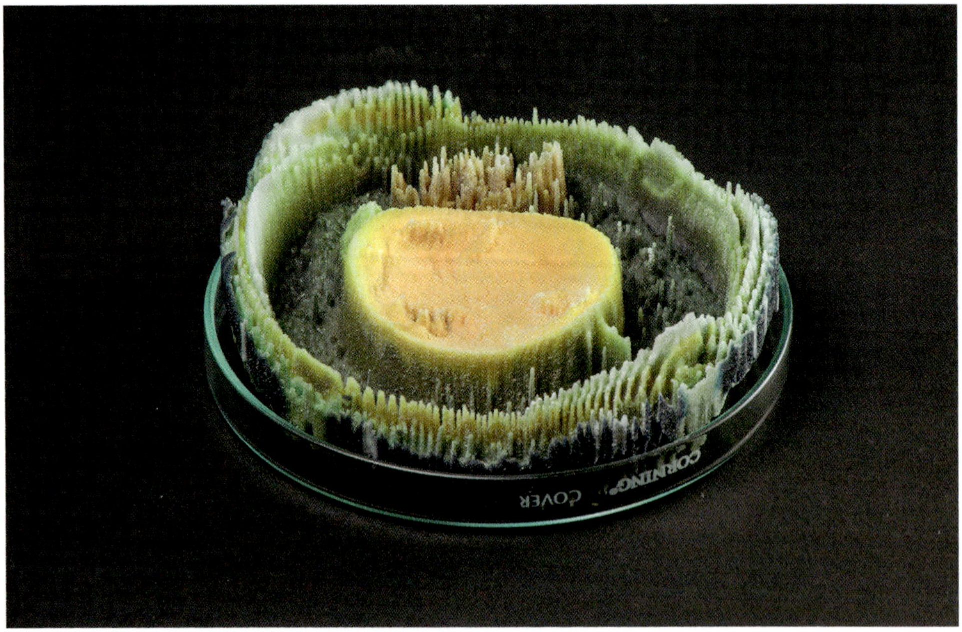

Figure 84. Suzanne Anker, *Remote Sensing #7*, 2013.
Plaster, pigment, resin, glass Petri dish, 4 x 4 x 2 in (10.15 x 10.15 x 5cm).

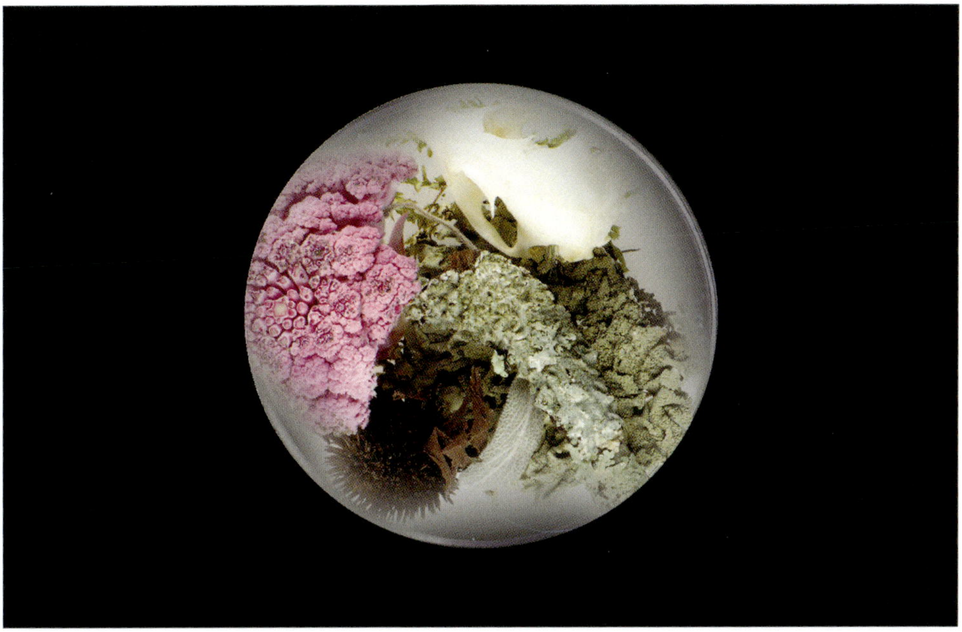

Figure 85. Suzanne Anker, *Vanitas (in a Petri Dish) #13*, 2013.
Archival inkjet print on paper, 42 x 42 in (107 x 107 cm).

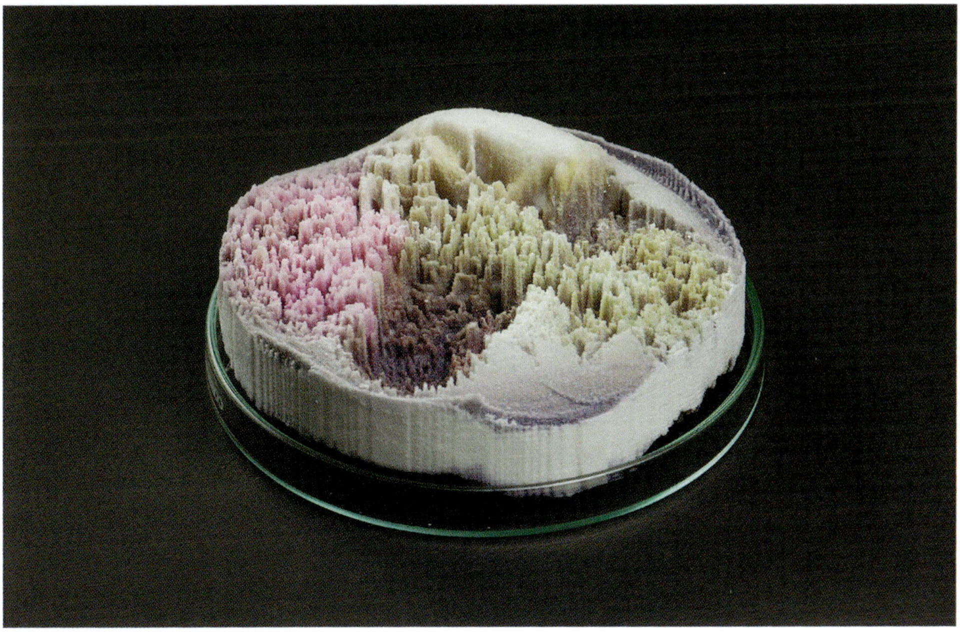

Figure 86. Suzanne Anker, *Remote Sensing #12*, 2013.
Plaster, pigment, resin, glass Petri dish, 4 x 4 x 2 in (10.15 x 10.15 x 5 cm).

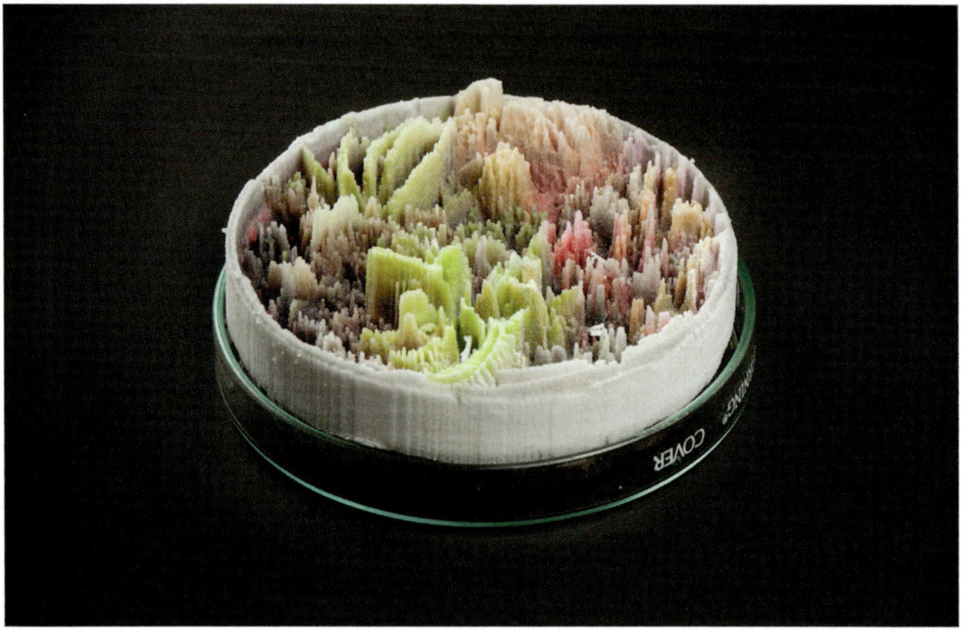

Figure 87. Suzanne Anker, *Remote Sensing #13*, 2013.
Plaster, pigment, resin, glass Petri dish, 4 x 4 x 2 in (10.15 x 10.15 x 5 cm).

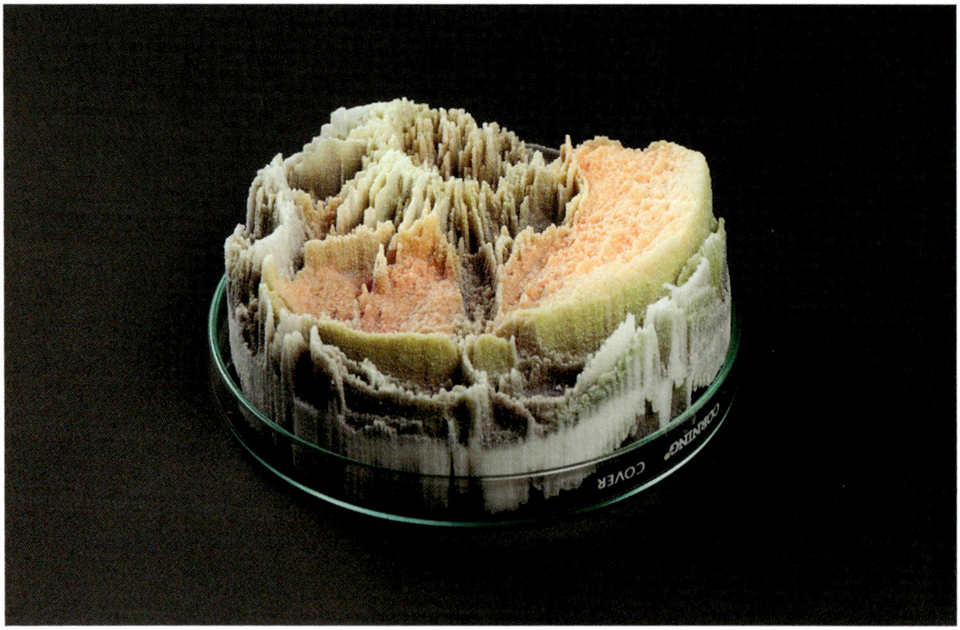

Figure 88. Suzanne Anker, *Remote Sensing #20*, 2013.
Plaster, pigment, resin, glass Petri dish, 4 x 4 x 2 in (10.15 x 10.15 x 5 cm).

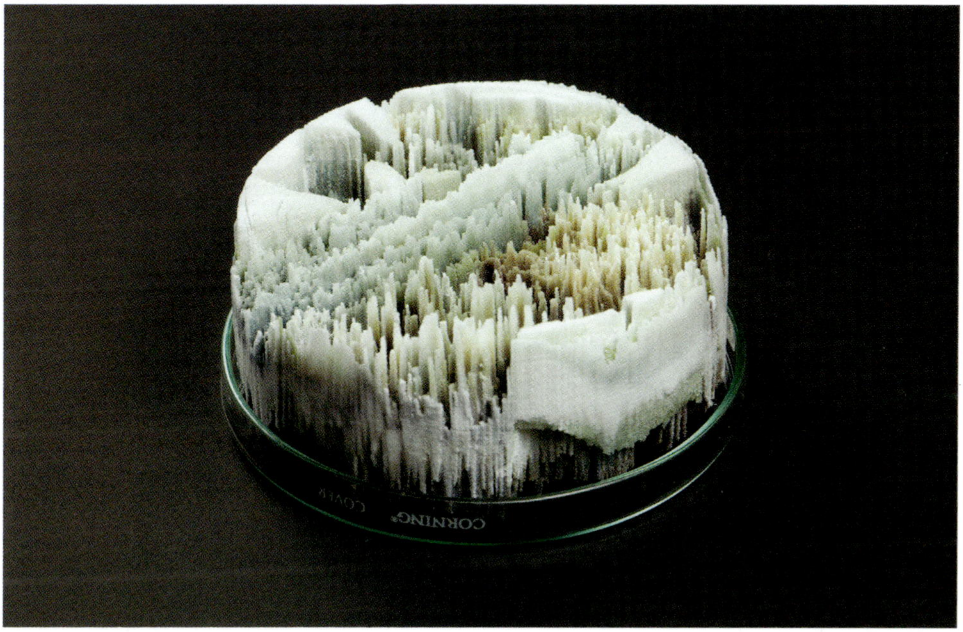

Figure 89. Suzanne Anker, *Remote Sensing #23*, 2013.
Plaster, pigment, resin, glass Petri dish, 4 x 4 x 2 in (10.15 x 10.15 x 5 cm).

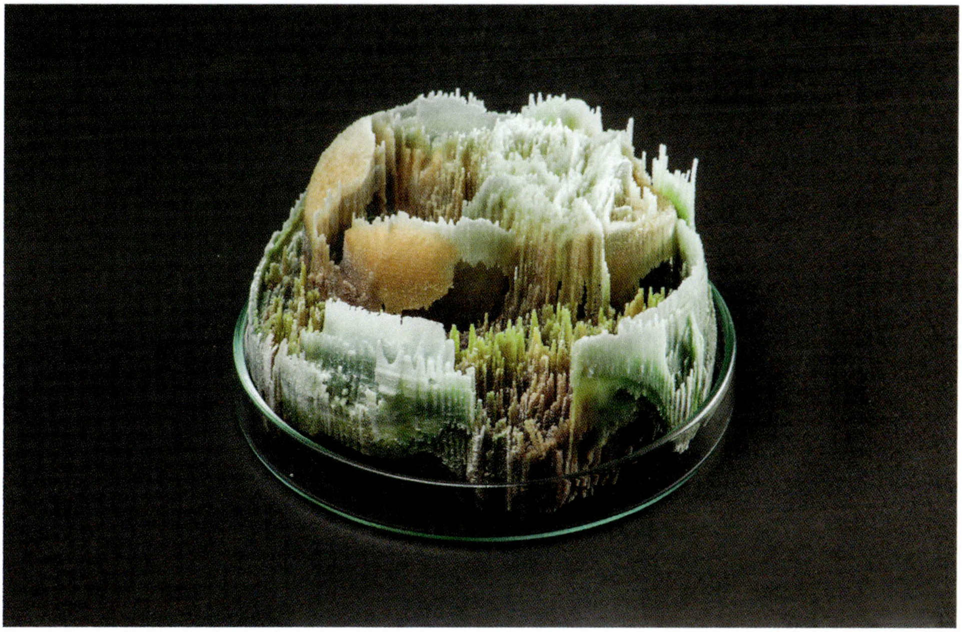

Figure 90. Suzanne Anker, *Remote Sensing #2*, 2013.
Plaster, pigment, resin, glass Petri dish, 4 x 4 x 2 in (10.15 x 10.15 x 5 cm).

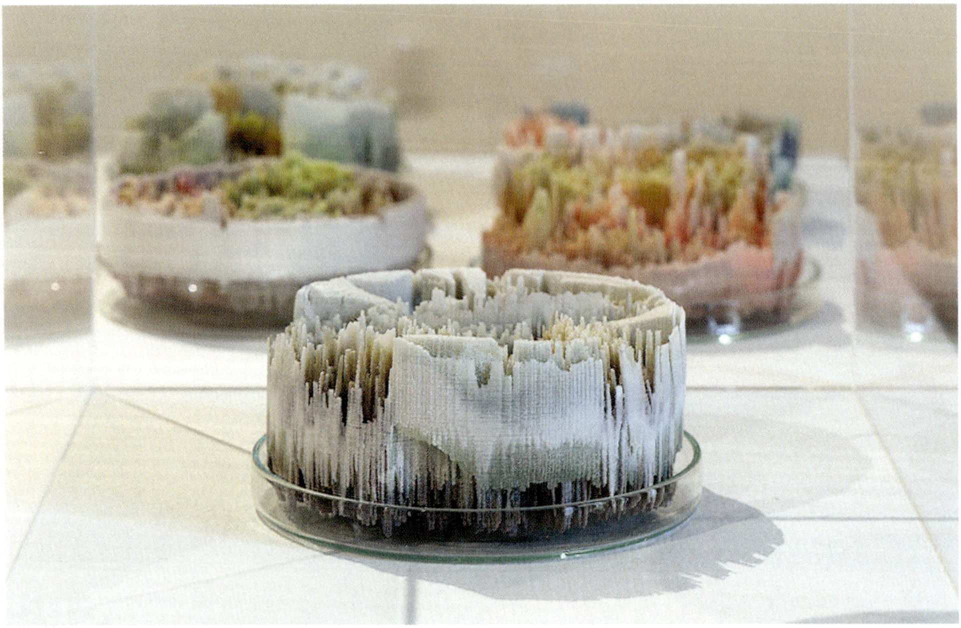

Figure 91. Suzanne Anker, *Remote Sensing* series, 2013. Plaster, pigment, resin, glass Petri dishes, 4 x 4 x 2 in (10.15 x 10.15 x 5.08 cm) each. Installation view at *Remote Sensing: Microlandscapes and Untold Stories* at Deborah Colton Gallery, Houston, Texas, 2014.

SF: Do the colors have particular significance? Are they chosen purposely? Are they related to any technical processes, to color theories?

SA: The pieces are about color "as is." Unlike painting, there is no mixing or tampering with pigments. Each object is burnished with color that is already a constituent element. Cherries, papaya, and pomegranates are saturated with red and orange. When I set up the *Vanitas* pieces, I generally look towards texture as well.

SF: What was your interest in transforming the photographs again into objects?

SA: I have always worked between two and three dimensions. Each transposition creates a novel way of seeing which, in turn, presents alternative significations. I was interested in seeing how a sign could be made to resemble its initial object or, in fact, alter it. Whereas the original object was in low relief, the fabricated sculpture heightened those coordinates of scale. In addition, the extrusion separated planes into peaks simulating the way crystals grow. Delicate parts of the sculpture were magically composed of a variety of colors in striated form. Such transfers from one form to another means of production is usually inventive since

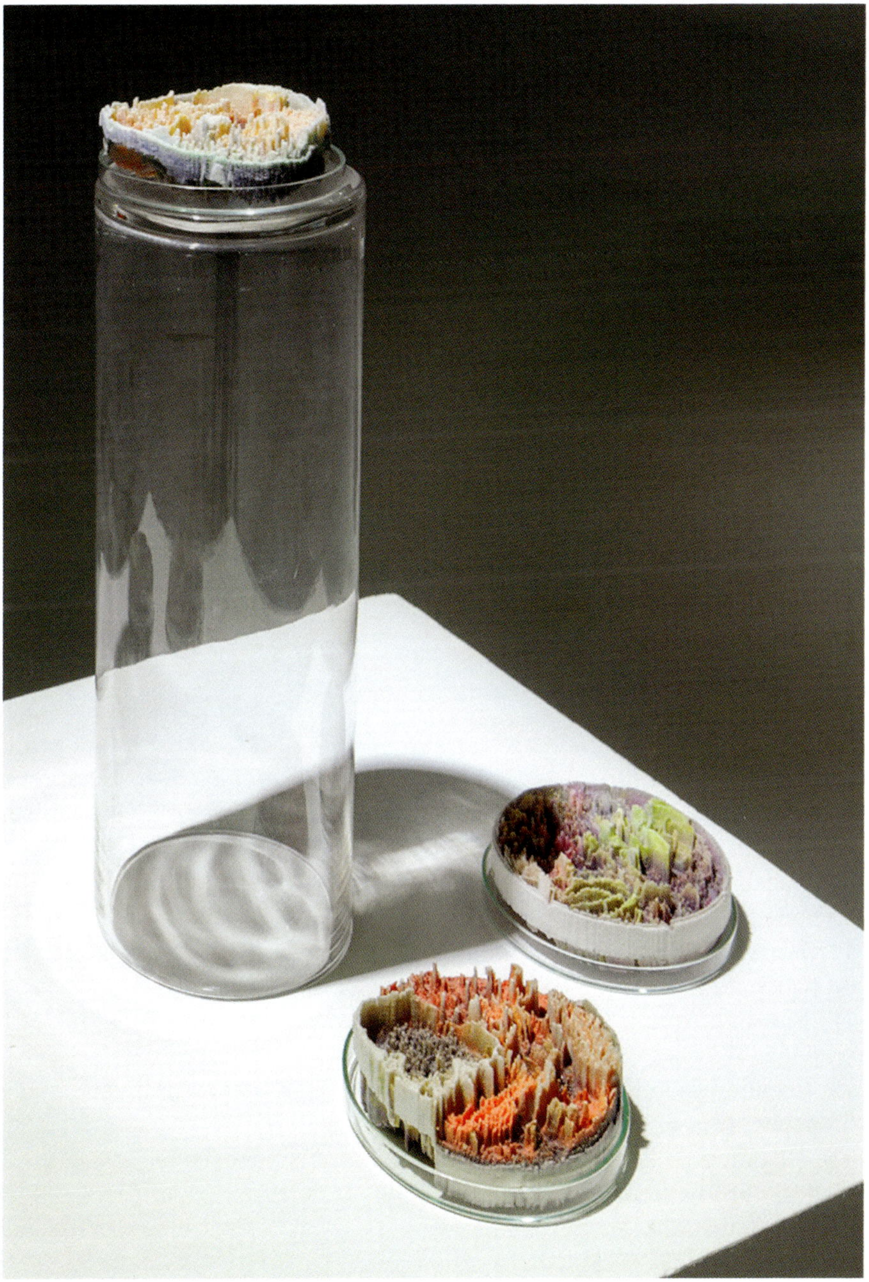

Figure 92. Suzanne Anker, *Remote Sensing* series, 2013.
Plaster, pigment, resin, glass Petri dish, glass tower. Left: 4 x 4 x 12 in (10.15 x 10.15 x 30.48 cm) Right: 4 x 4 x 2 in (10.15 x 10.15 x 5.08 cm) each. Installation view of *Rainbow Loom* at SNAP, Shanghai, China, 2014. Photograph by Henry G. Sanchez.

outcomes are not known. One might say that this process creates epistemic objects, as the theorist Hans-Jörg Rheinberger speculated, referring to knowledge producing artifacts. Microlandscapes are part of a new kind of map-making, a simulated geography constructed out of data. Here, data becomes material, forging relations between space and topography.

References

Buchloh, Benjamin H. D. "Farewell to an Identity." *Artforum* 51, no. 4 (2012): 252-263.

McKibben, Bill. *The End of Nature*. New York: Random House, 1989.

Rheinberger, Hans-Jörg. *Toward a History of Epistemic Things: Synthesizing Proteins in the Test Tube*. Stanford, California: Stanford University Press, 1997.

List of Illustrations

Fig. 75: Suzanne Anker, *Vanitas (in a Petri Dish)* series, 2013. Inkjet prints on paper mounted on board, 42 x 42 in (107 x 107 cm) each. Installation view of *Rainbow Loom* at V Art Center, M50 Creative Garden Shanghai, China, 2014. Photograph by Henry G. Sanchez.

Fig. 76: Suzanne Anker, *Vanitas (in a Petri Dish) #8*, 2013. Archival inkjet print on paper, 42 x 42 in (107 x 107 cm).

Fig. 77: Suzanne Anker, *Vanitas (in a Petri Dish) #3*, 2013. Archival inkjet print on paper, 42 x 42 in (107 x 107 cm).

Fig. 78: Suzanne Anker, *Vanitas (in a Petri Dish) #2*, 2013. Archival inkjet print on paper, 42 x 42 in (107 x 107 cm).

Fig. 79: Suzanne Anker, *Vanitas (in a Petri Dish) #15*, 2013. Archival inkjet print on paper, 42 x 42 in (107 x 107 cm).

Fig. 80: Suzanne Anker, *Rainbow Loom*, 2014. Wooden table, 366 glass Petri dishes, various items collected in China, 36 x 192 x 36 in (91.4 x 487.7 x 91.4 cm). Installation view of *Rainbow Loom* at V Art Center, M50 Creative Garden Shanghai, China, 2014. Photograph by Henry G. Sanchez.

Fig. 81: Suzanne Anker, *Rainbow Loom*, 2014. Wooden table, 366 glass Petri dishes, various items collected in China, 36 x 192 x 36 in (91.4 x 487.7 x 91.4 cm). Installation view of *Rainbow Loom* at V Art Center, M50 Creative Garden Shanghai, China, 2014. Photograph by Henry G. Sanchez.

Fig. 82: Suzanne Anker, *Petri's Panoply*, 2014. Wooden table, 186 glass Petri dishes, various items collected in Germany, 36 x 96 x 36 in (91.4 x 244 x 91.4 cm). Installation view of *[macro]biologies II: organisms* at Art Laboratory, Berlin, 2014. Photograph by Suzanne Anker.
Fig. 83: Suzanne Anker, *Vanitas (in a Petri Dish) #1*, 2013. Archival inkjet print on paper, 42 x 42 in (107 x 107 cm).
Fig. 84: Suzanne Anker, *Remote Sensing #7*, 2013. Plaster, pigment, resin, glass Petri dish, 4 x 4 x 2 in (10.15 x 10.15 x 5 cm).
Fig. 85: Suzanne Anker, *Vanitas (in a Petri Dish) #13*, 2013. Archival inkjet print on paper, 42 x 42 in (107 x 107 cm).
Fig. 86: Suzanne Anker, *Remote Sensing #12*, 2013. Plaster, pigment, resin, glass Petri dish, 4 x 4 x 2 in (10.15 x 10.15 x 5 cm).
Fig. 87: Suzanne Anker, *Remote Sensing #13*, 2013. Plaster, pigment, resin, glass Petri dish, 4 x 4 x 2 in (10.15 x 10.15 x 5 cm).
Fig. 88: Suzanne Anker, *Remote Sensing #20*, 2013. Plaster, pigment, resin, glass Petri dish, 4 x 4 x 2 in (10.15 x 10.15 x 5 cm).
Fig. 89: Suzanne Anker, *Remote Sensing #23*, 2013. Plaster, pigment, resin, glass Petri dish, 4 x 4 x 2 in (10.15 x 10.15 x 5 cm).
Fig. 90: Suzanne Anker, *Remote Sensing #2*, 2013. Plaster, pigment, resin, glass Petri dish, 4 x 4 x 2 in (10.15 x 10.15 x 5 cm).
Fig. 91: Suzanne Anker, *Remote Sensing* series, 2013. Plaster, pigment, resin, glass Petri dish, 4 x 4 x 2 in (10.15 x 10.15 x 5.08 cm) each. Installation view at *Remote Sensing: Microlandscapes and Untold Stories* at Deborah Colton Gallery, Houston, Texas, 2014.
Fig. 92: Suzanne Anker, *Remote Sensing* series, 2013. Plaster, pigment, resin, glass Petri dish, glass tower. Left: 4 x 4 x 12 in (10.15 x 10.15 x 30.48 cm) Right: 4 x 4 x 2 in (10.15 x 10.15 x 5.08 cm) each. Installation view of Rainbow Loom at SNAP, Shanghai, China, 2014. Photograph by Henry G. Sanchez.

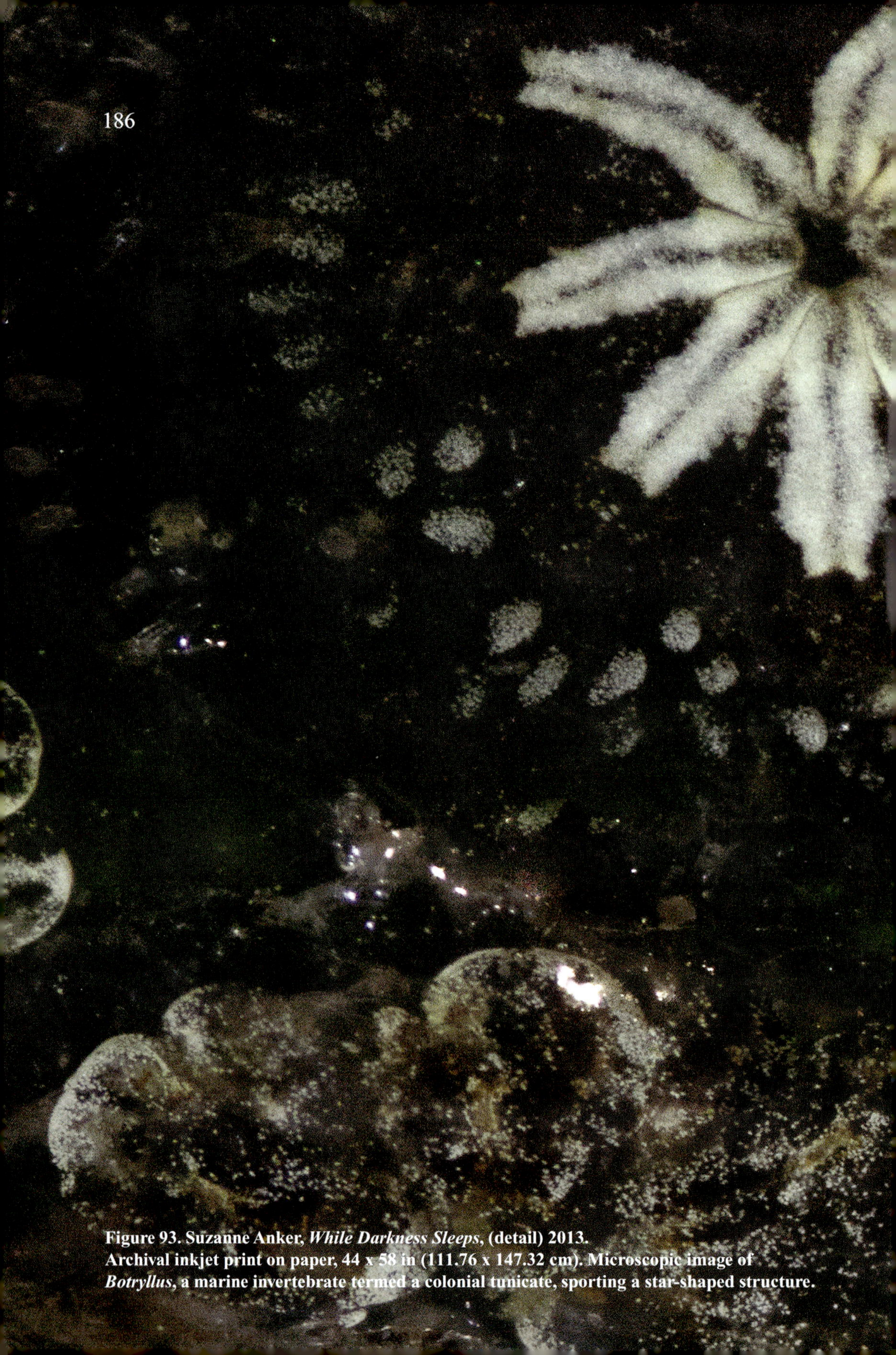

Figure 93. Suzanne Anker, *While Darkness Sleeps*, (detail) 2013.
Archival inkjet print on paper, 44 x 58 in (111.76 x 147.32 cm). Microscopic image of *Botryllus*, a marine invertebrate termed a colonial tunicate, sporting a star-shaped structure.

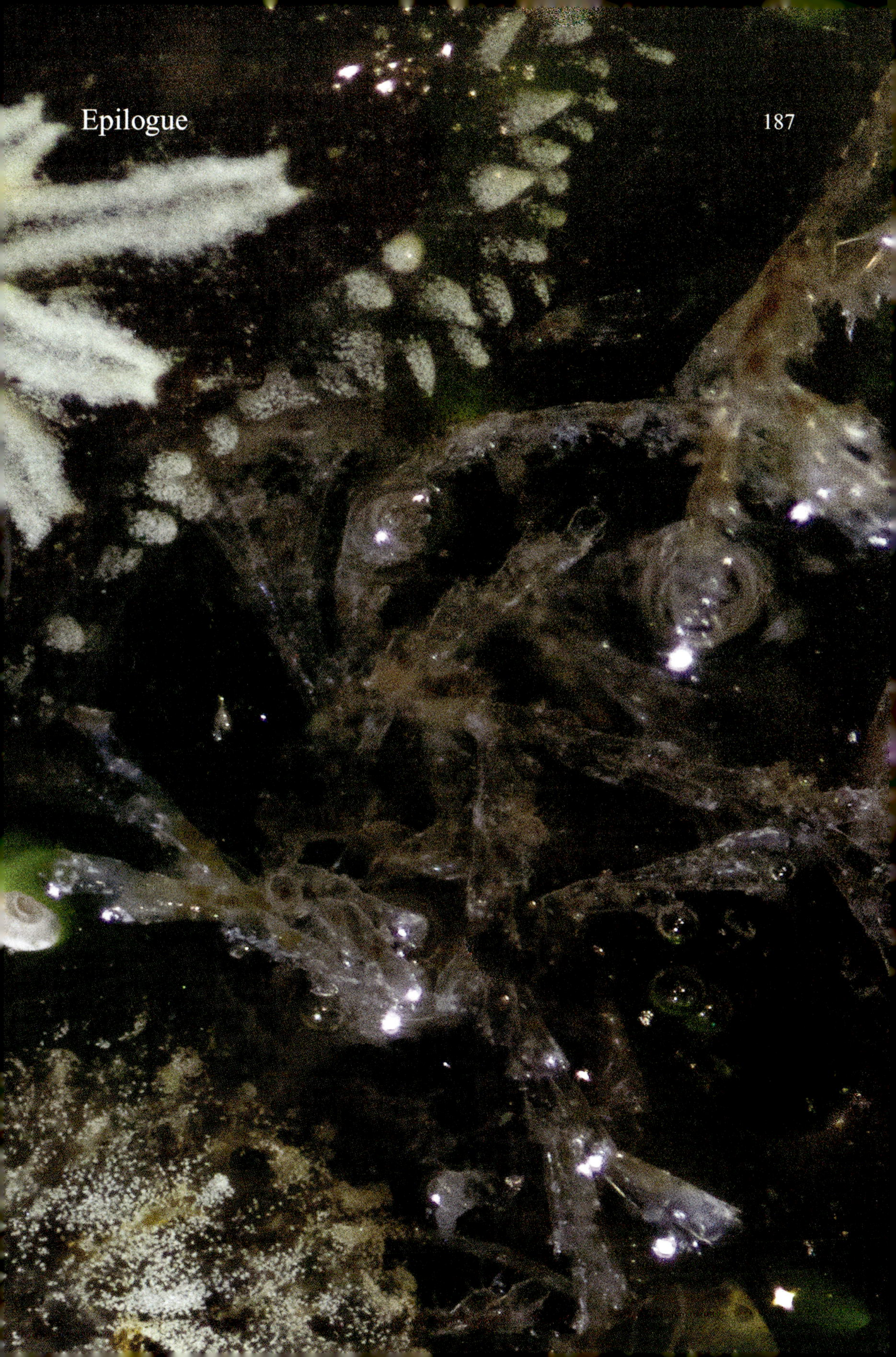

Epilogue

Suzanne Anker & Sabine Flach

Sabine Flach: SVA's Bio Art Laboratory in your Fine Arts Department at the School of Visual Arts in New York City is quite unique. What was the impetus behind the decision to incorporate a Bio Art Laboratory into your program? There are very few, if any, Bio Art labs in the world that reside in art schools. Obviously, you are at the forefront of this directive. Where would you position your Bio Lab in regard to visual art?

Suzanne Anker: Art has always been connected to nature. From the Paleolithic cave paintings and Venus statuettes, through Romanticism and the biomorphic forties, the natural world has always functioned as a source of inspiration for artists. Genres such as the still life, portrait, and landscape also find their sources in nature. More recently, earth works, video and performance art as well as eco art can be cited. SVA's Bio Art Lab is a state-of-the-art laboratory where students are introduced to the tools of science as additional ways to produce art. Employing microscopic images in photography (fig. 93), painting with fluorescent bacteria and algae, tissue culturing of plants and deciphering DNA are some of the projects that have evolved.

SF: Outcomes of such practices connect Bio Art to contemporary trends in Bio Design and Bio Architecture. It seems to me that artists, as well as scientists, often use this term in a naïve way. What is Bio Art and where are its connections to biology?

SA: Since the late 1980s many artists have turned their attention to working with biologically related concepts and materials. Of course the infusion of biology into the visual arts is not new in itself. For art critic Jack Burnham, a discrete change in art took place in the late sixties, not because it was a heeded proclamation by Arthur Danto that art was over, but because the visual arts began to partner with seminal processes and create alternative methodologies connected to art practice: earth works, systems theory and real-time media became new working tools for artists. As early as 1969, in *Beyond Modern Sculpture*, Burnham sees the integration of "men and machines into optimally functioning systems as tantamount to

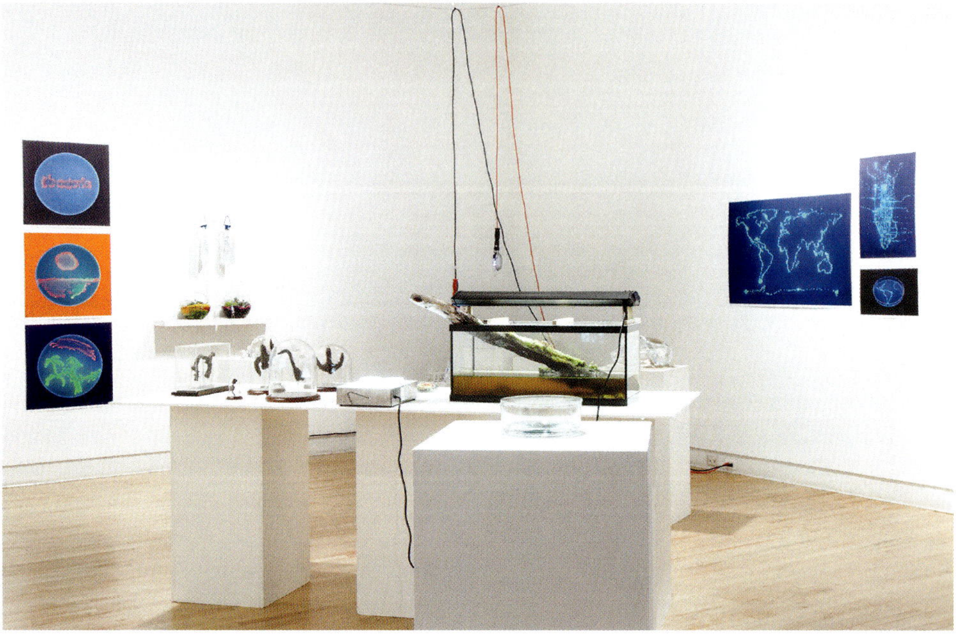

Figure 94. Installation view of *Where is the Art in Bio Art?*, curated by Suzanne Anker, SVA Flatiron Gallery, 2014. The exhibition included photographs of bacteria paintings (left and right walls), terrariums, contaminated soil sculptures, Petri dishes, and a stained and cleared specimen. Photograph by Beatriz Meseguer.

creating synthetic organisms."[1] It is synthetic biology today that has captured the imagination of artists, designers and scientists as a new molecular tool intended to transform matter and its attendant theoretical concerns. What is novel is the adaptation and exploitation of biologically-generated art which harnesses the advanced developments in technical apparatuses, making visible or statistically believable what has never been accounted for before.

Let us begin with a working definition of Bio Art,[2] a contested term in itself (fig. 94). In dissecting this genre of art, three distinct yet sometimes overlapping subcategories emerge. These subgenres take into consideration the allied epistemic practices necessary to transform matter on a molecular level. First various artworks emerged portraying the iconography of instrumentalized–visionMRI scans, the Atomic Force Microscope, electrophoresis, and PCR technologies among others. Images of chromosomes and their genotypic and phenotypic vari-

1 Jack Burnham, *Beyond Modern Sculpture: the Effects of Science and Technology on the Sculpture of this Century* (New York: George Braziller, 1975), 54.

2 See Suzanne, Anker, "The Beginnings and the Ends of Bio Art," *Bio Art: Life in the Anthropocene, Artlink* 34, no. 3 (2014): 14-15.

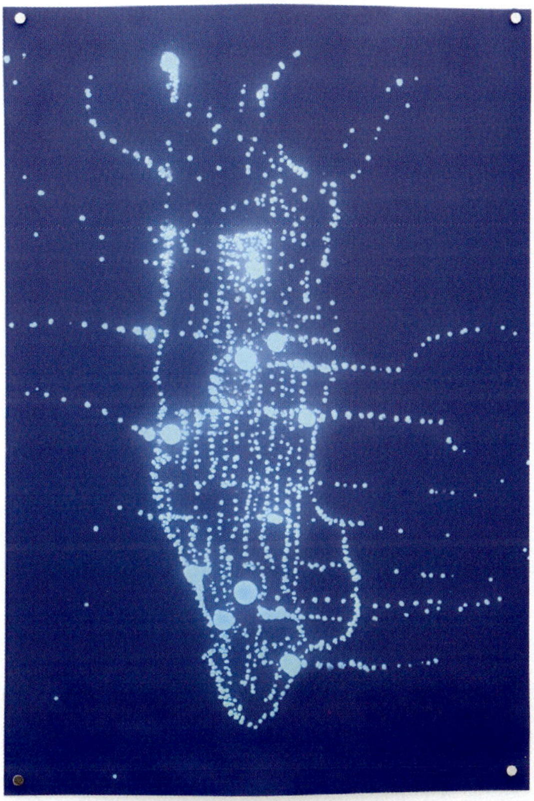

Figure 95. Lina Espinosa, *Manhattan*, 2013. Fluorescent bacteria painting. Archival inkjet print, 17 x 26 in (43.2 x 66.04 cm). Photograph by Raul Valverde.

ations in animals and plants appeared in various artists work. Some of these images operated as cultural critiques of science while others document genetic mutations of insects, resulting from nuclear radiation. Additionally full body scans, pictures derived through sonograms and images of laboratory fabricated animals entered into the domain of culture, be it painting, sculpture, photography, video, music, theater as well as their popular culture variants.

Secondly, the incorporation of 3D modeling software, systems theory, artificial life, robotics, biodegradable scaffolding and an interest in emergent theories of life became a source of techniques and subject matter. New media installations, rapid prototype sculptures and algorithmic code writing became tools for producing art, as photography and video had previously incorporated novel technologies into visual art.

And thirdly, most certainly the integration of wet laboratory practices such as tissue engineering, the cloning of plants, and transgenic microorganisms became subject matter and materials employed by artists. Lina Espinosa and Yacov Avrahami have worked with these materials. In the former, the artist has composed a subway map of Manhattan in New York City in fluorescent bacteria (fig. 95). Avrahami's work simulates watercolor but is in fact a bacteria landscape (fig. 96).

Living matter as an art-making medium, brought many artists into scientific laboratories to work with scientists through collaborative residency programs, particularly in Europe and Australia. Like canaries in a mine, artists-in-labs became a spark for innovation and controversy.

Of particular importance to Bio Art is to summon awareness of the political, economic and social consequences of altering life. From relational aesthetics to performance art, from the institutional critique to new media installations, from photographic realities to manipulated ones, Bio Art is supported by these and other platforms. Scientific paraphernalia, biological processes, body fluids and serums often accompany this work. And frequently dead or live animals, plants, and microorganisms accompany the work as well. It is most common to see charts, sensors and computer chips as part of this engagement (fig. 98).

As a cross between art and science, design and architecture, what parameters are in place to evaluate Bio Art? Various works operate on a sliding scale between the end points of art and science. Can a work of Bio Art be judged based on the difficulty of biological processes being employed? Are Bio Artists no more than amateur scientists? Can the philosophical questions Bio Art may ask be embedded in visual art scenarios or do design principles come in to save the day: hand-blown glass, lab coats as costumes, arrays of plants and horticulture apparatuses, robotic systems, etc. Can Bio Art be separated from Bio Design? What is the role of utility in these manifestations? These queries and more are some of the critiques concerning Bio Art.

SF: Although current trends in art have concentrated on appropriation and popular culture there seems to be an increase in the number of artists turning towards the natural world. Is Bio Art's infusion with the natural world a more current manifestation of Romanticism? A Neo-Romanticism?

SA: Whereas in the 19th century, Romanticism and Symbolism underscored a return to the landscape and the "self" as forms of secular spirituality and psychological mystery, Bio Art is dependent on and incorporated into technological processes. As a turn towards the natural world as a force expanding on Enlightenment principles, the Romantics were keen on uncovering the inner forces of human expression and agency. Art historical trajectories connecting the current state of Bio Art with past movements in art is a critical one, and in need of substantial discourse. Art criticism on its own is not well poised to critique this international movement, since many critics are not familiar with the materials and processes

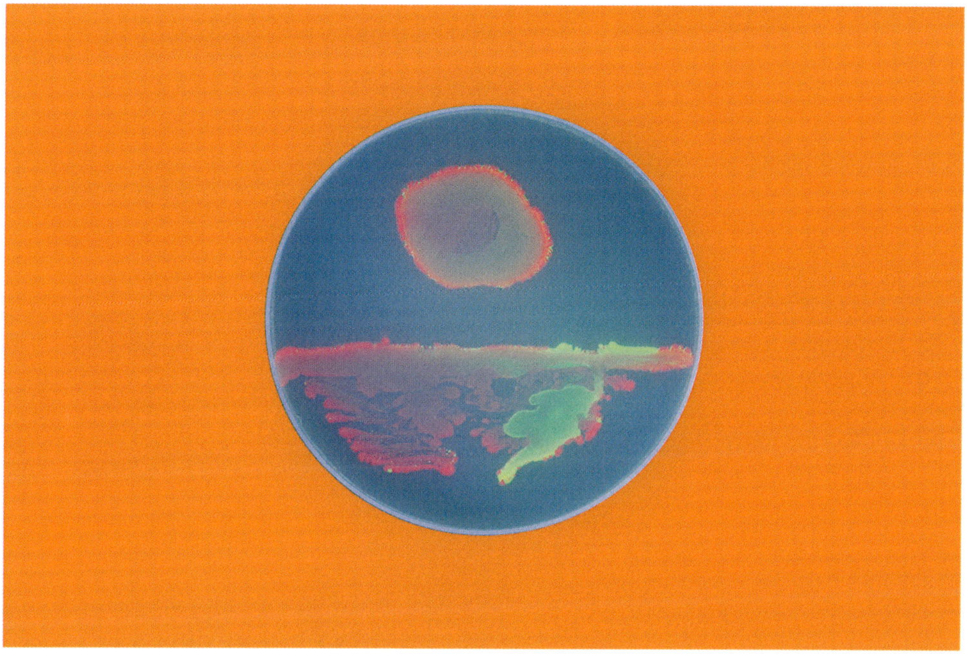

Figure 96. Yacov Avrahami, fluorescent bacteria painting, 2013.
Archival inkjet print, 44 x 30 in (111.76 x 76.2 cm). Photograph by Raul Valverde.

employed to create these works.[3] Bio Art's relation to the history of art as well as science, philosophy, anthropology and medicine, among others, make it a truly interdisciplinary practice.

SF: Would you say that Bio Art has the same kind of critical undertone and provocative attitude as Romantic art originally had?

SA: Although Romanticism and Bio Art share an equally diverse geographic distribution, Bio Art remains a subgenre of transdisciplinary practice. As a possible extension of Romanticism, one of its aims is to locate the "nature of nature" within the 21st century. And of course many of the works in this genre are extremely provocative, particularly in the area of performance.

SF: The Romantic era highlighted subjective experience. Would you say that this is relevant for contemporary Bio Art art as well?

3 See Michael Kimmelman's review of *Paradise Now: Picturing the Genetic Revolution* (2000), at Exit Art. Also see Eleanor Heartney, ed., *Art & Today*, Phaidon, 2013.

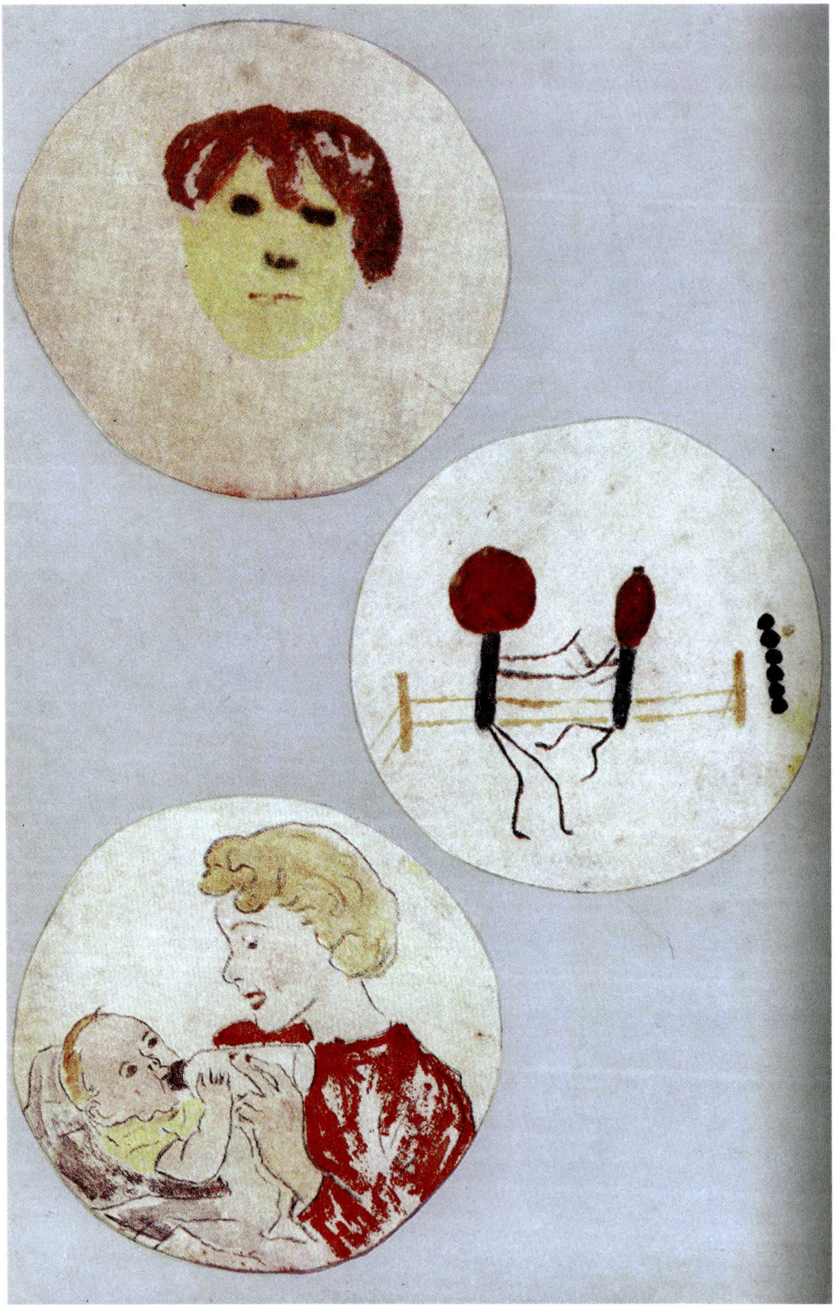

Figure 97. Bacteria painting by Alexander Fleming.
Courtesy: Alexander Fleming Laboratory Museum (Imperial College Healthcare NHS Trust).

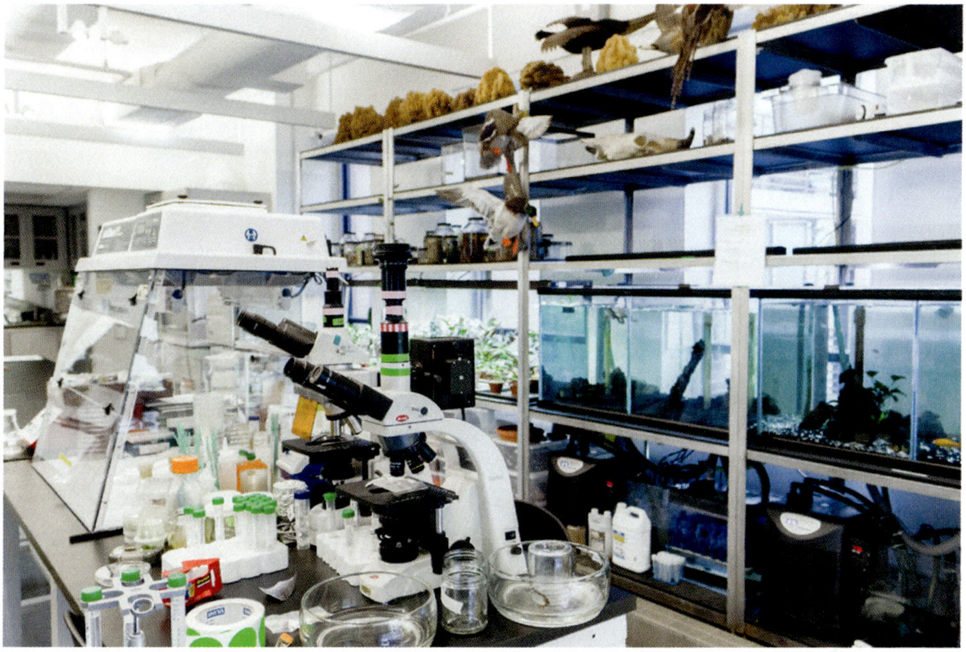

Figure 98. School of Visual Art's Bio Art Lab is a cross between 19th and 21st century biological laboratories. Housing animals and plants, as well as molecular reagents, the laboratory is a hybrid space where visual artists mix the familiar with the exploratory. Photograph by Raul Valverde.

SA: It is not the subjective experience that is the focus of Bio Art. It is the fusion of the imaginary with the analytical, the molecular with its phenotypical expression. The subtleties involved with the recognition in an experimental project is both cognitive and intuitive. Alexander Fleming, the father of penicillin, is a good example of this conjunction. His bacteria paintings were composed of different strains of microbes, producing colorful images in Petri dishes (fig.97).

SF: And emotions? The place of emotions, feelings and atmospheres played a significant role in the era of the Romantic. Is that relevant for your work?

SA: Not really. My interest in science is its distancing mechanisms. To embed myself into nature itself would result in sentimentality. Science's cold rationality imparts the possibility of criticality. However, art as an intersubjective experience oscillates between the senses, aesthetics and reason. Many contemporary practitioners are harnessing aspects of nature as it relates to current cultural transformations, whether in the realm of social critique, as in the works of Mark Dion, or Pierre Huyghe's installations incorporating aquariums as sites of splendor or Olaf Eliasson's waterfalls and light pieces. These kinds of work operate within the complexities of a global world in flux. The Anthropocene, a term suggested by scientist Paul Crutzen,[4] refers to geological distress impacting the Earth, resulting from human interventions into nature. He describes Earth's future as being rife with pollution and extinctions in which weather patterns will be largely disruptive to our food sources, infrastructures and life as we know it. He cites persistent waste, synthetic chemicals, and the acidification of coral reefs among Earth's contaminations.

More recently, public science writer Diane Ackerman has entered the debate in her current book, *The Human Age: The World Shaped By Us*. She considers "humans the most successful invasives of all time." Unlike many dystopian scenarios concerning the future, Ackerman is relying on human innovation to fix this condition: "We are dreamsmiths and wonderworkers. What a marvel we've become, a species with planetwide powers and breathtaking gifts."[5]

On the other side, however, environmentalist writer Rob Nixon, reviewing Ackerman's book for the New York Times is troubled by the "recklessness and greed" of companies who "have generated two-thirds of humanity's CO^2 emissions." [66] He also cites that "85 of the world's wealthiest individuals had a net worth equal to that of our planet's 3.5 billion poorest people."

I would just like to say that art is an experience, an inquiry, a commodity and a proposition about the world. Bio Art is well poised to explore and comment on the current condition of the world, either through the cultural imaginary or with living matter.

4 Paul J. Crutzen and Christian Schwägerl "Living in the Anthropocene: Toward a New Global Ethos." *Yale Environment 360*. January 24, 2011.

5 Diane Ackerman, *The Human Age: The World Shaped by Us* (New York: W. W. Norton & Company, 2014).

6 Rob Nixon, "Future Footprints," Book Review, *New York Times*, September 7, 2014, BR10.

References

Ackerman, Diane. *The Human Age: The World Shaped by Us*. New York: W. W. Norton & Company, 2014.

Anker, Suzanne "The Beginnings and the Ends of Bio Art." *Bio Art: Life in the Anthropocene, Artlink* 34, no. 3 (2014): 14-15.

Burnham, Jack. *Beyond Modern Sculpture: the Effects of Science and Technology on the Sculpture of this Century*. New York: George Braziller, 1975.

Crutzen, Paul J., and Christian Schwägerl. "Living in the Anthropocene: Toward a New Global Ethos." *Yale Environment 360*. January 24, 2011. http://e360.yale.edu/feature/living_in_the_anthropocene_toward_a_new_global_ethos/2363/.

Dunn, Rob "Painting With Penicillin: Alexander Fleming's Germ Art." Smithsonian Magazine online, July, 2011 Heartney, Eleanor, ed. *Art & Today*, Phaidon, 2013.

Heiferman, Marvin, and Carole Kismaric. *Paradise Now: Picturing the Genetic Revolution*. Saratoga Springs, NY: Tang Teaching Museum and Art Gallery, Skidmore College, 2001.

Kimmelman, Michael. "Art in Review: Paradise Now." *The New York Times*, September 15, 2000. http://www.nytimes.com/2000/09/15/arts/art-in-review-paradise-now.html.

Nixon, Rob. "Future Footprints." Sunday Book Review. *The New York Times*, September 7, 2014, BR10.

List of Illustrations

Fig. 93: Suzanne Anker, *While Darkness Sleeps*, 2013. Archival inkjet print on paper, 44 x 58 in (111.76 x 147.32 cm).

Fig. 94: Installation view of *Where is the Art in Bio Art?*, curated by Suzanne Anker, Flatiron Gallery, School of Visual Arts, 2014. Photograph by Beatriz Meseguer.

Fig. 95: Lina Espinosa, *Manhattan*, 2013. Inkjet print of fluorescent bacteria painting. 17 x 26 in (43.2 x 66 cm). Photograph by Raul Valverde.

Fig. 96. Yacov Avrahami, fluorescent bacteria painting, 2013. Archival inkjet print, 44 x 30 in (111.76 x 76.2 cm). Photograph by Raul Valverde.

Fig. 97: Alexander Fleming's microbial art. Courtesy: Alexander Fleming Laboratory Museum (Imperial College Healthcare NHS Trust).

Fig. 98: School of Visual Art's Bio Art Laboratory, Fine Arts Department. Photograph by Raul Valverde.

3. Appendix

Mendell's Meltdown[1]

SUZANNE ANKER

When we think of natural history, or the *Origin of Species,* Charles Darwin takes flush and unabridged patrilineage. On the other hand, to whom or *what* do we grace with our co-evolved unnatural history, a saga of hereditary linkage incorporating, and tampered by, illusory manipulative strategies? This biological matrix is seduced, sautéed and sanctioned by reason as its main ingredient. Genetic engineering can be looked at as a colloidal mixture, suspending the commodification of the body with cyberreal ethics, where *Frankenstein* and *The Terminator* become the glorified residua of the cerebral imagination. In the name of fusion, we aptly combine seductive libidinal drive with its presumedly non-toxic mathematical and rhetorical other. Through the logic of biotech's genetic engineering, and reprotech's amnesia of ethical purpose, the reordering and redesigning of the future is figured in the ratio of even odds, speedily usurping destiny's arrow for the perennial game of crapshoot. From transgenic species to germline alterations, from bio-rhythmic (dis)proportions, to anti-Classical taxonomies, we are being taken for more than a bit of a spin. Do we really need cigarettes that glow in the dark?[2]

For the artist, in contrast to the scientist, a chromosome is a little figure, a hair-like finger-puppet hard-wired to the species. A chromosome becomes "colored body," whose name is derived from the laboratory technique of cell staining to reveal genetic matter under the microscope's lens. When a chromosome is disassembled or broken down into its prime molecular units, it can be read as a series of gene sequences, a printout that behaves and germinates as a code. In genetic design, one of the architectural coordinates of DNA is a sugar. A sugar, always present in genetic sequencing, forms the basis of our heredity and thus part of

1 Gregor Mendel was a 19th century scientist and monk whose work with pea plants led to the discovery of genetics. As a pun, his name in this text carries with it two L's, denoting scientists' capability to alter genetic code.

2 Dr. David Ow and his colleagues fused the genetic material of a firefly and a tobacco plant, forming glow-in-the-dark plants. David Ow et al. "Transient and Stable Expression of the Firefly Luciferase Gene in Plant Cells and Transgenic Plants." *Science* 234 (1986): 856-859.

our prime body language.[3] Each gene segment, like individual sugar crystals, is unique, and defines the particular properties within a singular species.

What is in question here implies the construction of the individual, in contradistinction to the formulation of the "self." Gene patterns may denote personalized cryptogrammic markers, but society and its institutions forge and fabricate the person. Simultaneously identity politics achieve a formal status of predeterminist theories, while biological destinies proliferate. These molecular programs form the flip side of governing social contracts. We continue to link biology with property and trade status, reinforcing social Darwinism in the name of progress. This practice of eugenics is very American, pragmatic but hardly Emersonian. Statistical analysis and its determining cachet has turned the war-machine into the gene-machine. Unsatisfied greed has no boundary.

With the discovery of radioactivity sub-atomic particles became powerful. Through nanotechnology, cells sports great value. The abject, dead, diseased or discarded were once disenfranchised specimens. This market-price protoplasm, now garnered as alchemical *confit,* even pales Warhol's drama of the necrophiliac. The factory *becomes* the body, as evidenced by America's glorification of materialism. With a three-hundred-sixty-degree turn, syndicated flesh industries are not only cannibalizing culture, but pimping nature itself. The cannibal, once thought of as a primal mishap of savage drive, greets us at the doorstep of corporate headquarters: Life Inc., Essential Biologicals, IVF America, Bionetics Foundation, to name a few. These family names like those before us, are merely calcifications of neomort mining.[4]

Body-part farms are industrial complexes, plantations functioning synchronously as host & parasite, terrorist & healer, garbage collector & soothsayer: a map in which the part and the whole occupy the same ethical stature. If we are fools for love (or power) are we not also game for the stalk? Can we think of ourselves as a collection of redeemable body-parts? Is it not the case when we co-author evolution? Through technofetishism, synthetic extensions parlay definitions of life, death and sexuality into a continuum requiring difficult assessment. In modernity, space can be radically separated

3 DNA and RNA usually occur in nature as macromolecules composed of smaller building block molecules called nucleotides. Each nucleotide consists of a 5-carbon sugar attached to a phosphate group and one of four nitrogenous bases, A, G, C and T. See Peter Russell, *Genetics*, 2nd ed. (New York: HarperCollins, 1990), 264.

4 "A 'brain dead' *neomort* refers to a warm, respirating, pulsating, evacuating, and excreting body requiring nursing, dietary, and general grooming attention" states Allan Turner. Through technological machinery, the *neomort's* organs are kept fresh for transplantation. Turner, Allan. "The Politics Of Death: Thirty-Nine Years and Counting." http://allanturner.com/death04.html. See also Andrew Kimbrell, *The Human Body Shop: The Engineering and Marketing of Life* (New York: HarperCollins, 1993), 38.

from time, repositioned, disembedded. This collage sensibility, not unlike the film edit, radicalizes our sense of doubt and interrupts our sagacity of the real. Genetic splicing using mechanical reproductive techniques has produced creatures such as Onco Mouse, Harvard II, and the Geep. With investigative paradigms shifting from chaos to complexity, the line between non-organic life and living systems can no longer be described as fixed, but instead as "phylic mechanism"[5] As we envision the future as code, impulse, chemical landscape or code within a code, we further abstract our vision and consciousness. Is there anything natural about history?

This essay was originally published in the exhibition catalogue *NaturKunden* (1993), Paszti-Bott Gallery, Cologne, Germany,

List of references

Darwin, Charles, and Gillian Beer. *The Origin of Species*. Oxford: Oxford University Press, 1996.

De Landa, Manuel. "Non-Organic Life." In *Zone 6: Incorporations*, edited by Jonathan Crary and Sanford Kwinter, 128-167. New York: Zone Books, 1992.

Kimbrell, Andrew. *The Human Body Shop: The Engineering and Marketing of Life*. New York: HarperCollins, 1993.

Ow, David W., Keith V. Wood, Marlene Deluca, Jeffrey R. Wet, Donald R. Helinski, and Stephen H. Howell. "Transient and Stable Expression of the Firefly Luciferase Gene in Plant Cells and Transgenic Plants." *Science* 234 (1986): 856-859. doi:10.1126/science.234.4778.856

Russell, Peter. *Genetics*, 2nd ed. New York: HarperCollins, 1990.

Turner, Allan. "The Politics Of Death: Thirty-Nine Years and Counting." http://allanturner.com/death04.html.

---

5 For further explanation of this concept see Manuel de Landa, "Non-Organic Life." In *Zone 6: Incorporations*, ed. Jonathan Crary et al., (New York: Zone Books, 1992), 128-167.

Errata/Erotica

SUZANNE ANKER

> The battle over where the body starts and ends has of course extended to the issue of reproduction, substituting the right of the unborn for the born, in thc same awkward metonymic exchange that allows the phone sex hype to replace body with voice.
>
> Celeste Olalquiaga, *Megalopolis*

Whether decoding the fetishist's masquerade or simply acknowledging cross-dressing, the repositioning of anti-Oedipal sexual models as principles of pleasure have become critical devices towards establishing elasticity in the mind-body scenario. To stipulate that sexuality is a known set, an equation based on constant variables, is to fall prey to quantitative measurement, to the point of excess. Pleasure is a principle of play and exploitation, offering itself up as a recharge to subliminally consecrated drive, reprogramming its own recital in a soliloquy without end. Pleasure and its self-replicating agendas act out the release mechanisms under which our cognitive attention is kept and held erect. To view the pleasure-paradigm as a fractal of charged units, as an electrically coded process, is to conceive of the arena in which sexuality, desire, hunger and thirst, obsession, addiction, compulsion, excitement, terror, anxiety, and fear find themselves as rent controlled tenants.

Eroticism and seduction as part of sexuality cannot be separated from voyeurism and fetishism, from sensorial input and metonymic fragmentation. Deep within our *sexual* catalogue, a textual encodement portrays and registers drives. As prescriptive markers, the menu of sexual preferences in Western culture carries within it, like a morality play, Judeo-Christian dogma of the patriarchal Super-Ego. The diffusion between sexuality as biological sign and gender as cultural construction is an attempt to separate the verb from the noun. In what *lingua* do we speak? Substantively, sex stands for the division of the species and distinguishes the male from the female in structure and biological function. In the verb tense, sex is the act of coitus. I wish to present here some thoughts on sexuality by separating the biological code from its cultural manifestation. If sexual preferences are erogenous parameters of cultural identity, are they not therefore fashionable notations inherent in sexual style? Does style, to become fashion, appropriate desire for the body by privileging particular zones? Premium culture-specific territories of the body are indeed loci of sexual options and practices.

Inspired by Saussure's science of signs, Roland Barthes' analytical study *The Fashion System*[1] reveals structural meaning in an industry consciously intent on creating desire. Using Barthes' system as a methodological device, a model of erotic discourse can be articulated through simple forms of substitution. In the chapter "Variants of Existence," Barthes makes an inventory of the elements of fashion, a taxonomy I will transfer to the realm of sexuality. Barthes states: "Indeed, the substance of the variant can never be confused with the substance of the genera, for the one is material (a coat, a clip), while the other is always non-material (long/short, slit/unslit)."[2] If we substitute "a coat, a clip" for "a cock, a clit," the material, and leave unchallenged the non-material (long/ short, slit/unslit) we enter into a dialogue of eroticism embedded in fashion's nomenclature. It follows accordingly that a cock or a clit can be long or short, slit or unslit. The significance of this system lies in metaphor and its tropes, where fashion replicates attributes of the body, that is, sexuality. Such a typology regards sexuality not as biological system, but as cultural construct, a meta-language. Other Barthian variants include: variants of form, variants of fit, variants of movement, variants of weight and suppleness, and variants of measurement.

Variant of Measurement

One of the semiotic features of fashion is represented by measurement. If at times measurements in fashion seem to follow rules of congruence – the glove to the hand, the leotard to the body, surrogate skins – mismeasurement is meant to exaggerate, even ridicule, fetishize or frighten. On the other hand, within the scientific model, the variants of measurement are used to identify, qualify and quantify. Through the assessment of DNA's chromosomal material, the laboratory specimen becomes the site for sexual determination. In genetic sequencing lies the signature of the sexual sign: XX, the sign of the female, and XY, the sign for the male. What happens to this model when the sign is expanded to include XYY or XXX? The story of the XYY gained public attention for the first time at Richard Speck's trial in Chicago[3]. In defense of the murder of eight student nurses, his attorneys devised an argument based on genetic data. They argued that the pattern of two Y chromosomes, rather than the XY configuration, had hard-wired a behavior of intense

1 Barthes, Roland. *The Fashion System*. (Oakland, CA: University of California Press, 1990).
2 Ibid., 111.
3 Stephen Jay Gould, *The Mismeasure of Man* (New York: Norton, 1981), 143-145.

aggression. In other words, being super male, XYY, the guy just couldn't help it. This postulate attributes a biological basis for cultural performance, indicating an analytic correspondence between possible (mis)readings in sexual representation and their signs. If Y is male, then YY must be even more male.

We see cultural mismeasurement, as well, in the formation of the XXX. Whereas scientific literature designates the normal female as XX, popular linguistic usage of XXX refers to descriptions of the charged character contained within film or pornographic advertisement:[4]

Exotic Hot XXX Women
or
Live XXX Phone Sex
or
Live Hot XXX Women

Following this logic, if XX is female, then who or what is XXX? This rating meant to describe the most sexually charged may in fact be describing an entity that is not woman, but one that is outside "femaleness." As a category constructed by the male subject, the sign as XXX acts on its own accord to underscore linguistic and cultural encodement in the fashioning of the concept of "more femaleness." Such extension of the female sign creates a biological proposition of alterity, rather than addressing the subject of womanhood. If woman is XX, then who is XXX? Is this analogy merely coincidental or does it sub-textually invade the psychological space where assumptions drawn from the body are repositioned onto cultural constructs? One by-product of language which distorts, encodes and injects cultural meaning onto sexual cyphers is the creation of prismatic nominal monsters.

A scathing discussion of gender and sexual construction is presented by Valerie Solanas,' *SCUM Manifesto*. As quoted in *Female Perversions*[5], the male is assumed to be a biological accident. For instance, "The male Y gene is an incomplete female X gene; the male is an incomplete female, a walking abortion." Maleness is an organic deficiency. The only honest males are transvestites and drag queens for the central desire for every male is to grow into his true self by becoming a woman."[6] This mirror-image distortion of mismeasured bio-logic is an example of the transgression from the noun to the verb, a delirious intellectual slippage. Weaving through the labyrinth of bio-deterministic politics, we confront provisional networks of information and access, as identity is constructed from

4 Adult classifieds. *The Village Voice* (New York), October 20, 1992.

5 Louise J. Kaplan, *Female Perversions: The Temptations of Emma Bovary* (New York: Doubleday, 1991), 356-359.

6 Ibid., 357.

these externally operative forces. Unlike memory, which is centered in the brain, the identity of an individual cannot be situated within the biological complex. Whereas biologically deterministic mechanisms may explicate characteristics relating to the species, the concept of an individual can only be socially formulated. Whereas biological sexuality can be encoded within the parameters of scientific practice, the event of sexuality is an identity issue.

Variant of Movement

Another of Barthes' variants is the element of movement, which "animates the generality of the garment." Barthes considers movement a value engaged in "rising, upsweeping, hanging, plunging, falling, swaying." How does it happen that movement or locomotion as a characteristic of cellular reproduction can be read through gender-laden points of view? How is this encoded into the nature of sexuality via reproduction?

Egg Not Silent Partners In Conception

"A human egg cell does not idle languidly in the female reproductive tract, like some Sleeping Beauty waiting for sperm Prince Charming to come along and awaken it for fertilization. Instead, new research indicates that most eggs actively beckon to would-be partners, releasing an as-yet-unidentified chemical to lure sperms cells."[7] The scientific reproductive model traditionally casts the female egg as a passive receptor. However, if the egg does not passively lay in waiting, but instead signals her quarry "to swim towards the squirt of the fluid," this phenomenon engages female conception as an active participant. Such chemical attraction resets the biological dialogue in the mode of submission/domination collaboration. Magnetic and chemical attractors, operating as locomotive fields, alter assumptions regarding gender difference.

Eroticism is never without its entourage of change, decoys, allurements, stimulations, titillations and even pain. It's the private, decorous affair of the individual. Stimulating the appetite through deceit and glamour, our pleasure com-

7 Carol Ezzell, "Egg Not Silent Partners In Conception." *Science News* 139, no. 14 (1991).

plex fantasizes and recognizes what it wants to want. The origins of sexuality in the formation of the initial gamete retells the story of the violence from which we emerge: "The tense maneuvers between well-armed sperm and fortified egg echo back to the first moments when sexual reproduction evolved." Beginning with one-celled organisms, reproduction was merely a geometric affair...cloning, splitting, dividing. However, some small highly mobile cells, propelled by their search for the food nucleus, interlocked their DNA with the DNA of their targets. The newly formed organism now had a variable combination of genes and two parents. Thus the scenario of the origination of sexual reproduction has, as its source, the will for food.[8] *Eat or be eaten*, cannibalistic desires appropriate the cultural field and parallel issues of original sexual modes as when the prey and the predator could no longer disconnect. Or is it magnetic attraction?

Amalgamated by the excess of reason, the body has become a political site of cultural articulation: repositioned, dissected, culturally coded and vanishing. One can still imagine, however, that deep within unfilled recesses, something private still escapes public scrutiny and that when all is resaid and redone, our imaginary mechanisms and auto-seduction can still be soothed and recharged by the subliminal dangers of the sexual nexus.

This essay was written in conjunction with my exhibition, *Errata/Erotica* (1992) at B4A Gallery, New York City.

List of references

Barthes, Roland. *The Fashion System*. Oakland, CA: University of California Press, 1990.

Ezzell, Carol. "Egg Not Silent Partners In Conception." *Science News* 139, no. 14 (1991).

Gould, Stephen Jay. *The Mismeasure of Man*. New York: Norton, 1981.

Kaplan, Louise J. *Female Perversions: The Temptations of Emma Bovary*. New York: Doubleday, 1991.

Olalquiaga, Celeste. *Megalopolis: Contemporary Cultural Sensibilities*. Minneapolis: University of Minnesota Press, 1992.

Small, Meredith F. "Sperm Wars: The Battle for Conception." *Discover* (1991): 48-53.

The Village Voice (New York), October 20, 1992.

8 Meredith F. Small, "Sperm Wars: The Battle for Conception." *Discover* (1991): 48-53.

Synthetic Abandon

SUZANNE ANKER

> If nature represents a principle of economy, then culture surely must exemplify the principle of innovation through excess. When habits consume us, when our devotion to them exceeds the culturally defined norms, we label them as obsessions.
>
> Terence McKenna

For the automaton, to have a life of one's own is to be driven by a program…as each disk is implanted the robotic machine performs its act *sans* doubt or ambivalence. As an apparatus, the device appears as a body in the realm of control, a harmonious constituent, singular within its mechanism. Automatic behavior in an individual, however, interlopes with the obsessional: "The girl just can't help it," "Only one more time," "I'll stop tomorrow," "Just a little while longer." Sensory excess, memory and techno-mythic dreams create the signals from which obsession takes its cue, engineering programs of preoccupied will, advancing as a series of short circuits. Desire, fulfilling mastermind dreams, not unlike automata, is a drive stimulated by reason, while behaving as a harbinger of delight mixed with deceit. Desire brings with it post-mechanical intoxicants and the necessary injection of subliminal and physical avowals.

Injection, subjection, obsession, excess… terms of technology, terms of addiction. Pleasure centers, signals, receptors, cortical spasms, endorphins, metabolites, stimulants, depressants, rhapsodics, inhalants… ringers for the high… the fix… the orgasmic engagement with encoded Dionysian markers. If violence is a necessity to nature, is ferocity inherent to natural form? And what about the power of the machine? Not of free will, but of necessity, an essentialist ingredient in the status of the program. The pleasure/pain principle so readily apparent in our organic process becomes inescapably a component of our machine… our fantasy… our fetish of the will. We give up control under the illusion of an ever-perfected-easier-than-thou-dream-mix of future plenty. Giving up control through pleasure and anodynes creates the sequence: pleasure/pain/pleasure/pain/pleasure/pain… a score orchestrated with operatic additives, conjugal spare parts, and pharmacological regalia, eagerly at work metabolizing entropy. Automatism. Automatism as machine, automatism as a post-hypnotic theater. Somnambulism. Self-exploitation through expansion. Phantasmagoria. The fetish.

Alfred Binet's analysis of the fetish as an "enchanted object" that mysteriously held sway over individual destiny[1], chromatically resonates with the relentless agency inherent in human chromosomes. Fetishism can be linked with addiction in Binet's own terms which parallel the "posture of submission (*assujetissement*) to fetishistic paradigms of idolatry and idealization."[2] This posture of submission, the way in which desire overcomes the "self," is operative in both addiction and creation. The nineteenth century brought the hypodermic syringe as apodictic tool for cultural procreation, a modernist instrument of evolutionary exchange. Our invention of ever more efficient painkilling devices provides even greater degrees of post-mechanical-pain. The suppressant implicates the perpetrator in seductive complicity. We already had from the eighteenth century the cabinet and its secret contents. That is, as defined in the *Encyclopedia*, a private place, a divide, a room in which the secret fetish could be housed.[3] Could not such a fetish be a pill, a liquor case, a candy box, a paint set or even a studio? The *potentia* of secrecy unveiled is the modality of a cabinet, where desire runs as frenzy, on the gasoline of fantasy.

Fantasy is our double agent, a rhapsody of dreamy neurons in collision with each other unfolding as a process of consciousness. Overstimulated, overeager to cash in, over bombarded with phantasmagoric delight, such consciousness, unlocalized, induces corporeal denial. In *Megalopolis*, Celeste Olalquiaga talks about the suspension of self in technological society: "Fulfilled by a compulsive repetition that ultimately saturates the libidinal need, pleasure is contained precisely where conventional reality and simulacra become indistinguishable; compulsion acts itself out in the form of rituals.[4]" Like automata, the contemporary body is thought of in terms of its fragmentation; our compulsions and obsessions are interchangeable as mutable sectors. Excessive desires, hubris, the colonization of pleasure centers by technological compulsions have driven our desires to a soaring pitch. Whether symptomatic of current technological anxiety or part and parcel of genetic forbearing, our sugar-based nucleotide sequences continue to lust for another sweet tooth.

1 Emily S. Apter, *Feminizing the Fetish: Psychoanalysis and Narrative Obsession in Turn-of-the-Century France* (Ithaca: Cornell University Press, 1991), 20.

2 Ibid., 21.

3 Emily Apter quotes Hubert Damisch's "The Museum Device: Notes on Institutional Changes." *Lotus International* 35 (1982): 5. For further discussion see Apter's essay "Cabinet Secrets: Peep Shows, Prostitution, and Bric-a-bracomania in the Fin-de-siecle Interior." In *Feminizing the Fetish: Psychoanalysis and Narrative Obsession in Turn-of-the-Century France* (Ithaca: Cornell University Press, 1991).

4 Celeste Olalquiaga, "Reach Out and Touch Someone." In *Megalopolis: Contemporary Cultural Sensibilities* (Minneapolis: University of Minnesota Press, 1992), 6.

This essay was originally published in the exhibition catalogue *Art Addicts* (1992) at V-Space, New York City.

List of references

Apter, Emily S. *Feminizing the Fetish: Psychoanalysis and Narrative Obsession in Turn-of-the-Century France*. Ithaca: Cornell University Press, 1991.

Apter, Emily S. "Cabinet Secrets: Peep Shows, Prostitution, and Bric-a-braco-mania in the Fin-de-siecle Interior." In *Feminizing the Fetish: Psychoanalysis and Narrative Obsession in Turn-of-the-Century France*. Ithaca: Cornell University Press, 1991.

Hubert, Damisch. "The Museum Device: Notes on Institutional Changes." *Lotus International* 35 (1982): 4-35.

McKenna, Terence. *Food of the Gods: The Search for the Original Tree of Knowledge A Radical History of Plants, Drugs, and Human Evolution*. New York: Bantam, 1992.

Olalquiaga, Celeste. "Reach Out and Touch Someone." In *Megalopolis: Contemporary Cultural Sensibilities*. Minneapolis: University of Minnesota Press, 1992.

Viruses and Pearls: The Materialization of Culture

SUZANNE ANKER

The onslaught of viruses and their strategies have in a sense taken over the work of the unconscious.

Jean Baudrillard

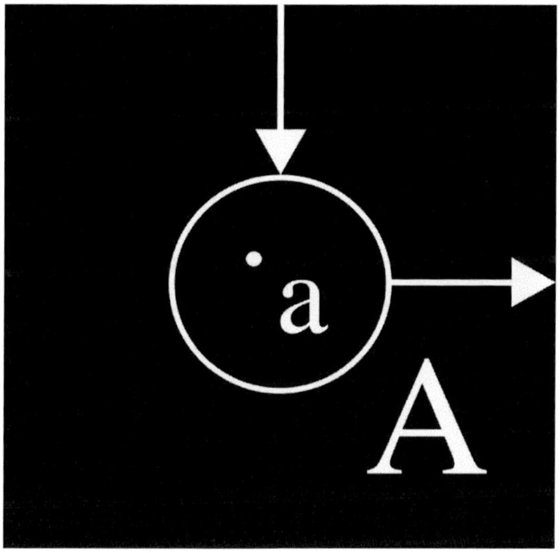

Figure 99. In order to accomplish a critical fiction the functions of 'a' as subset and 'A' as matrix are self-reflexive.

Cryptograms and hyperfictions, cybersex and smart drugs, transpecies germlines, body-part-commodities... cultural buzzwords, all hovering in the media, encoding with its signature the information eruption of the cyborg and the technofix. From the metacognitive to the manic, from the substitutive to the social, codes have become our operative conductor. Our all and nothing mind material, haptically deciphering the complexities of the constructed world. Within this network *what* is culture? What is its composition? As an integrated and conglomerate pattern of human knowledge culture is comprised of history, the biological and physical sciences, anthropology, psychology, mathematics, poetry, geography, philosophy, visual art et al. It is the sum total of activity recorded and reflected upon (produced, experienced and consumed) through a penetration with natural and artificial domains. As a subset of culture, art is a single species, a way of knowing the world through illusion or fiction, an imaginary infatigable narrative. However, art also functions simultaneously as a matrix, giving its subject the diagnostic ability of a paradox – the paradox of *critical fiction* (fig. 99).

What is the substance of 20th century art if not the texts of the whole culture, of other disciplines? By engaging perception, metaphor and material judgment in its formulations, art enjoins the building of the cultural body. As a matrix it gives actuality to metaphorical thinking, using as its database the entirety of cultural history. For the Minimalists and their specific objects, metaphor emerged from phenomenology and perception. For the Pop practitioners, the semiotics of late industrial society was an aligning subject. And for the Surrealists, the nature of the unconscious became a targeted sanctuary. How can such subjective experiences or manifestations based in illusion be part of reality, part of cognitive history? It is precisely through a position of criticality in fiction that art does accomplish this paramount task.

To culture living material under artificial conditions transmutes matter into living forms of, say, viruses or pearls. Biologically-based-cultural-production creates raw data for scientific experimentation, producing molecular recipes and analytic enzymes. Does human culture operate in a parallel way? Is it possible to employ biological metaphors to decipher aesthetic or cultural relations? This sociobiological line of thought proposes a molecular politic, one operative in the construction of cultural paradigms. Richard Dawkins, in particular, discusses the relationship of natural evolution to cultural evolution. He cites the *meme*[1]:

> A meme is a unit of cultural transmission, or a unit of imitation. Examples of memes are units, ideas, catch-phrases, clothes fashions, ways of making pots or building arches. Just as genes propagate themselves in the gene pool by leaping from body to body via sperm or eggs, so memes propagate themselves in the meme pool by leaping from brain to brain via a process which in the broad sense can be called imitation.

The use of argument based on metaphor may be quite convincing, but when does its analogical value contort its proportions? While Dawkins' meme theory may propose a parallel relationship (gene : gene pool as meme : meme pool), is this correlation really anything more than a structural convenience? Are these ratios equivalent? Whereas, the organization of the part to the whole may be acknowledged as a coextensive form, this equation cannot be expanded to include behav-

1 Richard Dawkins, *The Selfish Gene* (Oxford: Oxford University Press, 1976).

ior, manifestation, actualization or even time. These are, in fact, the very faculties of human contingency. And by what genetic rule will phenotypes be actualized from this vast encoding process? If prediction was possible, as it is in Mendelian law, then how come the cultural world is not predictable? Driven by glamour factors, the cultural conglomerate continually breaks the surface tension of biological determinism in novel and unexpected ways. Whereas the gene can determine species *potentia* – and not behavior – the meme can only take into account the concepts of cultural consciousness. Neither prediction nor market manipulation can formulate the infinite varieties of cultural forms. One consequence of this line of reasoning sets up a molecular politic in which social and cultural theories encapsulate an anthropomorphized natural world. To metaphorically separate cultural theory from the body politic is one function of the precincts of art.

The virus is either a simple organism or a complex molecule – a parasite-like predator vagabonding for a home, a transitive postmodern body, incapable of its meta-status without its reliance on living cells, to be used as a translational system. The pearl, a synchronously abnormal growth – the result of an irritant or a virus – enters the establishment as a gem. Secretions giving form to entities is our reliance on culturing, on interchanging error with procreative capacity. Culturing has linked art production with other incorporations of foreign bodies – bodies of cognitive resources once thought to be outside the domain of visual art. Like a virus or a pearl, visual art is an altered mutation within this transformative epoch.

This essay originally appeared in *N.A.P. text(s)* 1, no. 2 (1995): 14-15.

List of references

Baudrillard, Jean. *The Transparency of Evil: Essays on Extreme Phenomena*, translated by James Benedict. London: Verso, 1993.

Dawkins, Richard. *The Selfish Gene*. Oxford: Oxford University Press, 1976.

List of illustrations

Fig. 99. Diagram created by Suzanne Anker in 1995 for the The National Academies Press.

Biographies

Suzanne Anker

Suzanne Anker is a visual artist and theorist working at the intersection of art and the biological sciences. She works in a variety of mediums ranging from digital sculpture and installation to large-scale photography to plants grown by LED lights. Her work has been shown both nationally and internationally in museums and galleries including the Walker Art Center, the Smithsonian Institute, the Phillips Collection, P.S.1 Museum, the JP Getty Museum, the Medizinhistorisches Museum der Charite in Berlin, the Center for Cultural Inquiry in Berlin, the Pera Museum in Istanbul, the Museum of Modern Art in Japan, and the International Biennial of Contemporary Art of Cartagena de Indias, Colombia. Her books include *The Molecular Gaze: Art in the Genetic Age*, co-authored with the late sociologist Dorothy Nelkin, published in 2004 by Cold Spring Harbor Laboratory Press, *Visual Culture and Bioscience*, co-published by University of Maryland and the National Academy of Sciences in Washington, D.C. Her writings have appeared in *Art and America, Seed Magazine, Nature Reviews Genetics, Art Journal, Tema Celeste and M/E/A/N/I/N/G.* Her work has been the subject of reviews and articles in the *New York Times, Artforum, Art in America, Flash Art,* and *Nature.* She has hosted twenty episodes of the *Bio Blurb* show, an Internet radio program originally on WPS1 Art Radio, in collaboration with MoMA in NYC, now archived on Alana Heiss' Art On Air http://artonair.org/series/the-bio-blurb-show. She has been a speaker at Harvard University, the Royal Society in London, Cambridge University, Yale University, the London School of Economics, the Max-Planck Institute, Universitiy of Leiden, the Hamburger Bahnhof Museum in Berlin, the Courtauld Institute of Art in London, Banff Art Center any many others. Chairing SVA's Fine Arts Department in NYC since 2005, Ms. Anker continues to interweave traditional and experimental media in her department's new digital initiative and the SVA Bio Art Lab. http://bioart.sva.edu

Sabine Flach

Prof. Dr. Sabine Flach is an art historian focusing on modern and contemporary art and theory, including interdisciplinary approaches to biology, psychology and the sciences of cognition. She is Chair of the Institute for Art History at the University of Graz, Austria, where she is currently Professor of Modern and Contemporary Art. She studied art history, theory of literature, philosophy and humanities in Marburg, Perugia, Kassel and Berlin, and has held teaching positions at TU Berlin, HU Berlin, University of Hamburg, University of Kassel, and Mills College in Oakland, California. From 2000 to 2010, she was head of the research department "WissensKünste–Art of Knowledge and Knowledge of Arts" at the Center for Literary and Cultural Studies in Berlin. Her recent book publications include: *Körper-Szenarien. Zum Verhältnis von Körper und Bild in Videoinstallationen*. München, published in 2003 by Wilhelm Fink; *Warburgs Denkraum. Formen, Motive, Materialien*. München published in 2014 by Wilhelm Fink, ed. Pablo Schneider and Martin Treml; *Darwin and Theories of Aesthetics and Cultural History*, published in London 2013 by Ashgate Publishing Company, ed. Barbara Larson; *WissensKünste. Die Kunst zu wissen und das Wissen der Kunst – WissensKünste.*, published by VDG Weimar in 2011, ed. Sigrid Weigel; *Habitus in Habitat III–Synaesthesia and Kinaesthetics*, published in Bern, New York 2011 by Peter Lang, ed. Jan Soeffner and Jörg Fingerhut; *Habitus in Habitat II–Other Sides of Cognition*, published in Bern, New York 2011 by Peter Lang, ed. Jan Soeffner; *Habitus in Habitat I – Emotion and Motion*, published in Bern, New York 2011 by Peter Lang. ed. with Daniel Margulies and Jan Soeffner. Her current research projects include: *Naturally Hypernatural–Contemporary Arts and the Relation to Nature*; *For Those Who Know–Artistic Knowledge and the Art to Know*; *Aesthetics, Aisthesis and Media of Embodiment*; *Epistemology and Aesthetics of Visual Thinking*; *Art between Scene and Scenario–New Concepts of Performance, Sculpture and Space in the Arts since 1960.*

Art / Knowledge / Theory

Edited by Suzanne Anker and Sabine Flach

Art / Knowledge / Theory is a book series that explores artistic modes of expression as forms of knowledge production. It focuses on transdisciplinary, epistemological and methodological approaches to contemporary art. Linking artistic and scienti¢ c practices, tools, techniques and theories, the volumes investigate the cultures of aesthetics and science studies as they relate to works of art.

Art / Knowledge / Theory analyzes the role of art in contemporary culture by probing the philosophical, historical and social parameters by which images are accessed and assessed.

As an amplification – as well as intervention or even a correction – to historical research, this series questions the state of the art and knowledge within a culture, characterized by technology and science.

Volume 1	Suzanne Anker, Sabine Flach (eds) Embodied Fantasies: From Awe to Artifice 2013, ISBN 978-3-0343-1102-1
Volume 2	Suzanne Anker, Sabine Flach The Glass Veil: Seven Adventures in Wonderland 2015, ISBN 978-3-0343-1101-4
Volume 3	Mika Elo, Miika Luoto (eds) Senses of Embodiment: Art, Technics, Media 2014, ISBN 978-3-0343-1233-2